P9-BIJ-795

The Doctor's Guide to

Tennis Elbow, Trick Knee, and Other
Miseries of the Weekend Athlete

The Doctor's Guide to
TENNIS ELBOW,
TRICK KNEE,
AND OTHER MISERIES
OF THE
WEEKEND ATHLETE

BY
Leon Root, M.D.
AND
Thomas Kiernan

David McKay Company, Inc.
NEW YORK

THE DOCTOR'S GUIDE TO
TENNIS ELBOW, TRICK KNEE, AND OTHER MISERIES
OF THE WEEKEND ATHLETE

Library of Congress Catalog Card Number: 74–82610

ISBN 0–679–50460–5

MANUFACTURED IN THE UNITED STATES OF AMERICA

Designed by Bob Antler

For Paula.
Doubly so.

AUTHOR'S NOTE

Although this book is the result of a full and complete collaboration between the two authors, it is written in the first-person-singular voice of Dr. Root to spare the reader any confusion of identities.

The reader should also note that the therapeutic exercises sprinkled throughout the book are designed to speed the rehabilitation of sports-related ailments and injuries and to reduce the possibility of their recurrence. Since *unsupervised* exercise is in itself capable of causing injury, these exercises should be approached with a certain amount of caution and a large measure of common sense. They should not be started until symptoms of acute inflammation and pain have subsided. Nor should they be undertaken by anyone in ill health unless he has his physician's permission.

New York

L.R.
T.K.

CONTENTS

1. Introduction   1
2. You, Your Sport, and Your Misery   8
3. You and Your Body   25
4. Your Elbow Miseries—Tennis Anyone?   56
5. Your Knee Miseries—Trick or Treat!   102
6. Your Back Miseries   155
7. Your Ankle Miseries   197
8. Your Shoulder Miseries   211
9. Your Hip Miseries   227
10. Your Wrist and Hand Miseries   238
11. Your Foot Miseries   251
12. Your Muscle Miseries   261
13. A Final Word   276
    Index   279

The Doctor's Guide to

Tennis Elbow, Trick Knee, and Other
Miseries of the Weekend Athlete

1

INTRODUCTION

The title tells the story of this book, so there is little need to engage in extensive preliminaries. What I am going to do in these pages is explain to you in plain, nontechnical English the whys and wherefores of the various ailments you suffer due to your leisure-time athletic activities, and how you can prevent these ailments from interfering with your enjoyment of sports.

I do not intend to scare you away from participating in your favorite sports. Quite the contrary, my intention is to encourage your interest and participation, and at the same time provide you with a guide by which you can indulge your love of a sport and not be frightened away from it because of some temporary or permanent physical ailment you might be suffering as a result of it. As in all things in life, there is no substitute

1

for knowledge. I believe that with some hard knowledge about your sports-connected ailment, you will be that much more capable of participating in your favorite athletic activities, and of enjoying yourself as well.

As an orthopedic surgeon, I specialize in the treatment of sports injuries and ailments, among other things. Life would certainly be much more agreeable if we could all play our favorite sports without having to worry about broken bones, ruptured tendons, joint inflammations, muscle tears, and the like. But life is a never-ending series of contrasts, and we all know too well that pleasure cannot exist without pain. Thus, although doctors would prefer never to have to treat patients whose ailments derive from so healthy and pleasurable an endeavor as sports participation, alas we must!

Yet, until very recently, it has been something of a tradition among physicians to look upon sports-related ailments with less than grave concern. One of the reasons for this is that, until recently, sports ailments were not as common as they are today; it has only been since the great sports-participation explosion of the early 1960s that doctors have found more and more of their patients coming to them with complaints that are the specific result of an athletic activity.

Another reason is that most doctors didn't know a great deal about the *psychology* of sports ailments. They generally treated them as they would any other affliction, neglecting to take into account the psychological effects such miseries were likely to have on their victims. If an individual stumbles over a curb on his way to work and severely wrenches his knee, he is probably glad of the few days of bed rest his doctor orders—it justifies his taking some time off from his job, enables him to catch up on his sleep and reading, and provides him with an opportunity to be waited on by his dutiful and sympathetic family.

However, if that same individual is a regular weekend touch-football or tennis player, say, and he wrenches his knee during the course of a game, he is going to be pretty unhappy about not being able to play his favorite sport for weeks or even months, and then only with reduced mobility and effectiveness.

This was basically the difference between the treatment of non-sports-associated and sports-associated ailments of the same general type. Until recently, doctors tended to approach them identically, without taking into account the differing motivations and needs of the individuals who suffered them. But with the appearance of a new branch of medicine called "sports medicine," the consciousness of many doctors is now being raised, and sports-connected injuries and ailments are receiving the special attention they deserve.

There are three fundamental ways in which the development of sports-medicine seems likely to benefit all of us weekend athletes—men and women alike. The first is its consideration of the psychological motivations of the victims of sports ailments: it understands that sports-minded people want to get better in a hurry so that they can return to their favorite activities.

The second derives from the first: the sports-medicine approach not only emphasizes normal healing, it also places great value on educating the sufferer in the ways and means of participating in his or her favorite sport *despite* the presence of an ailment. Usually these ways and means will include the hastening of healing through various pharmacological procedures and the specific strengthening of the area around which the ailment has occurred. It may also consist of elective corrective surgery when such surgery is indicated as being the best and quickest means of restoring an ailing body part and enabling the sufferer to return to his sport.

The third way in which the sports-medicine approach benefits all of us weekenders is closely related to the first two: in becoming a specialized branch of medicine, it has generated considerable research into sports-associated injuries and ailments. This in turn has given doctors new and better methods of treatment. It has also provided us with valuable information about the particular nature and incidence of sports ailments and about such important matters as the best equipment and clothing to use to reduce the chances of such disorders occurring or recurring.

This is not to suggest that we have learned all we need to know about athletic ailments. Far from it. Nevertheless, if you have a sports-connected problem (and you wouldn't have picked up this book if you didn't) and consult a doctor who has been exposed to sports medicine and its healing rationale, you are likely to find the treatment you receive considerably more sympathetic and comprehensive than you would have fifteen or twenty years ago.

This book is designed mainly for those of you who haven't had an opportunity to consult a sports-oriented physician about your ailment, and who profoundly wish to keep up your participation in the sport in which your ailment has proved so painful, restrictive, and otherwise frustrating and bedeviling. It is not intended to be a substitute for a visit to your doctor. Nor is its purpose to provide you with the ability to officially diagnose your or your friends' ailments. Medical diagnosis is both an art and a science. It is a function of professional physicians, not amateur athletes. So, like the lawyer who has a fool for a client, the person who attempts to diagnose his own symptoms has a fool for a doctor.

Notwithstanding this disclaimer—and I don't mean it to sound as stern as it probably does—there is a great deal you can usefully learn about your sports ailment or ailments. Such knowledge can only stand you in good stead. It is my purpose in the chapters that follow to impart at least some of that knowledge.

It is not unusual for doctors these days to be critical of their own profession, and in this regard I am no exception. My principal criticism of the medical profession is that too many physicians put too much emphasis on the treatment of particular symptoms and not enough on the whole patient. As a result, too many patients are lulled into believing that once their symptoms are relieved, they have no further responsibility to themselves. This psychology has operated especially strongly in the case of non-life-threatening diseases and ailments. Once an individual's pain or discomfort is eliminated, he or she generally returns to the same bad habits of hygiene that produced the disease or ailment in the first place. This is one reason why there is so much chronic disease and illness in this country. Patients must not only be relieved of symptoms, they must also be encouraged and taught to avoid the conditions that so often bring about recurrence.

This theme will run as a central thread throughout the book. "The fault, dear Brutus, is not in our stars, but in ourselves, that we are underlings," my favorite poet, Shakespeare, once wrote to illustrate the idea that we tend to look outside ourselves for the causes of our

miseries, when the proper place to look is within. If I
achieve nothing else in this book, providing you with
the motivation to understand and successfully manage
your sports ailment will be achievement enough.

As a physician, I am aware of one of the most frequent complaints heard from patients—that doctors
don't tell them anything about their ailments. Again, I
would tend to agree with this, although from fifteen
years of personal experience I understand how difficult
it is for busy doctors to take the time to sit their patients
down—especially those who are not suffering from serious disorders—and explain their ailments in detail from
A to Z. It is an impasse that has existed since time
immemorial between patients and their doctors, and it
is likely to get even worse as the supply of physicians
decreases and the patient population expands.

Thus, another purpose in writing this book is to
provide you with the information that you have probably been unable to get from your personal physician in
satisfying detail because of his overcrowded schedule.
If you suffer from tennis elbow, for instance, or from
chronic tendinitis, trick knee, or any other sports ailment, I know how anxious you are to learn all you can
about the nature of your problem and the way it affects
the various components of your anatomy. Car owners
often evince no curiosity about the various mechanical
functionings of their automobiles until some component breaks down. People tend to take the same attitude with respect to their bodies: it is only when something goes wrong somewhere that an individual
suddenly needs to know all about the part of his or her
anatomy where the breakdown has occurred. This is
perfectly understandable, and would even be com-
mendable if doctors could expect that imparting such

information would serve to prevent further break-downs. Usually they can't. Again, once patients' symptoms are relieved, they forget all the valuable information they've received. But sooner or later they are back in their doctor's office with the same disorder.

I mention this only because I believe that the principal function of medicine should be the prevention of illness. Therefore, this book is devoted as much to explaining prevention as it is to showing you how you can continue playing tennis despite your tennis elbow, how you can continue bowling despite your bowler's thumb, and how you can continue your golf despite your bunions, bursitis (golfer's hip), and backache.

I cannot promise to cure any of your ailments in these pages. What I can promise is that with careful study you will understand the nature (and possibly the causes) of your ailments, and will learn how to deal with them in all the ways you should to make your leisure-time sports activities as enjoyable as possible.

With these few prefatory remarks, I wish you happy reading and healthy weekend heroics.

2

YOU, YOUR SPORT, AND YOUR MISERY

Aside from being a physician experienced in the treatment of sports-related ailments, I also have a good deal of personal, painful experience with such ailments—as does my coauthor, Thomas Kiernan.

As a college football player I suffered a back injury which, because I ignored it once the initial pain went away, has haunted me ever since and has made my participation in my favorite weekend sports a sometime thing. It is only when I keep my disc-weary back supple and strong through a faithfully followed back-exercise program that I feel safe on a tennis or squash court. Even then I don't feel all that safe, yet I risk the recurrence of a painful and disabling back problem for the sake of the very vital exercise and pleasure tennis and squash provide me.

Coauthor Kiernan was also a college football player. Like me with my back, he suffered a series of severe knee injuries. One knee was at least partially restored through surgery. The other knee he ignored. Today, it is the anatomical equivalent of a loose and rusty gate hinge, and he never knows when it will "go out" on him. He has also carried around with him for the past ten years a case of annoying and oft-painful tennis elbow. Yet he plays tennis, football, basketball and half a dozen other sports—at some risk, to be sure, but with little fear about his knee or elbow. This is because he has assiduously strengthened the muscles around his faulty joints so that many of the stresses his favorite sports entail are taken up by these reinforced supportive structures.

WHY WE SHOULD ENGAGE IN ATHLETICS

I mention these two personal case histories because they illustrate several points worth making at the beginning of this book. The first is that a great many of us bring our sports-connected ailments with us out of our youth and into adulthood. This can be either good or bad. It is good when it has made us aware of our anatomical weaknesses and motivated us to strengthen them so that they don't materially interfere with our enjoyment of sports and exercise. It is bad when its message has gone unheeded, and we continue to engage in activities that only further compromise or intensify our weakness—to the point where it becomes a severely chronic and often disabling condition.

The second point is that no matter what our particular sports-associated debility might be, it need not prevent us from participating in our favorite sports. Competitive sports and other athletic activities have a way of keeping us young—I don't mean cosmetically young, but organically young—and anything that performs such a service should be sought with gusto. Our hearts, our respiratory and circulatory systems, our gastrointestinal tracts, our reproductive functions, indeed, our very minds, are enhanced by sensible and regular exercise.

Now we all know that daily exercises of the calisthenic or setting-up variety can be quite boring and dissatisfying, and although every doctor is absolutely right to recommend them, he knows if he is at all realistic that few people possess the motivation and self-discipline to stick to them. That is why sports participation has so many attractions—it provides anticipation, excitement, and satisfactions that can never be achieved in the psychological and physical drudgery of the "daily dozen." Whether the sport is a competitive one, such as tennis or touch football, or a solo one, such as downhill skiing or long-distance running, it gives the participant a sense of joy and challenge, a healthy drive to extend him- or herself, and usually a complete body-workout that is far superior to ordinary setting-up exercises.

But we don't participate in sports primarily out of a concern for exercise. The very challenges and satisfactions I mentioned above, along with our taste for competition—either with others or with nature—get us out on the tennis court, ski slope or softball diamond. The camaraderie, the feel of the wind in our face, the pump of adrenaline through our system, the exhaustion of our energies, and the countless other sensual and psychological factors, all motivate us. The physical-health aspect is only a by-product of such drives.

That's precisely what is so delightful about sports: they fulfill the need for exercise without becoming a chore. The element of chore—of routine and repetition —in our lives tends to dull our senses and our minds. The old Greek dictum that a sound mind requires a sound body is a well-worn cliché, but it is a cliché precisely because it has proved so true through the centuries. When Socrates enunciated it, he was not talking about setting-up exercises but about the vigorous participation in athletic activities which not only challenge the body but also rejuvenate the mind with the satisfaction and sense of achievement the perfection of athletic skills provides.

I am certainly not discouraging the pursuit of daily setting-up exercises. They *are* effective for the maintenance of muscle tone and body line. Nevertheless, individuals who limit themselves to such calisthenics— when more provocative and challenging forms of exercise are available—are not gaining a tenth of the physical- and mental-health benefits they could achieve by pursuing a fairly strenuous sport, even if only on a weekend basis.

Of course, not all clichés are clichés because they're true. Many are accepted as true, but are in fact no truer than the myths that underlie them. One such myth is the popular contention that "no exercise is better than once-a-week or sporadic exercise." This is demonstrably false when it is applied to persons whose vital physiological functions are in a reasonably good state of health. I would certainly not recommend—no doctor would—that a person with a weak heart, or a heavy smoker, go out once a week and try to run five miles or play a furious game of full-court basketball. That would be potential homicide on the part of whomever made such a recom-

mendation, and probable suicide on the part of anyone who followed it.

However, for someone who is in fairly good physical condition and free of any organic weakness, a
strenuous session of tennis—or any athletic activity that
provides one with a healthy exhaustion suitable to one's
age and condition—once a week is far better than no
exercise at all.

A CAUTIONARY WORD

Of course, before anyone takes up a strenuous
sport—and even if one is currently involved in such a
sport—he or she should undergo a complete physical
examination to ensure that there are no physiological
or organic dangers involved in one's participation. I'm
not talking now about the common sports ailments en-
compassed by this book, but rather about heart and
vascular functions and other matters pertaining to the
vital organs, functions, and structures of the body. As-
suming that you pass such tests, you should then feel
free to pursue with gusto the sport or sports that most
satisfy you.

"Gusto" means just that. Each human body has its
own built-in defense mechanisms against overactivity
or total exhaustion, and except under a few circumstances your body will warn you when you are about to
overreach your capacities.

The most common exceptions relate to heat exhaustion, dehydration, and sunstroke, all of which can
act together to put you on your back before your body
has had a chance to adjust to the conditions that produce them. Thus, in addition to my caveat about having

a thorough physical examination, you should also have sense enough not to overextend yourself on a hot and humid day (more about this later).

One other frequent circumstance in which your body's warning system may not operate optimally is in the area of fatigue injuries to bones, ligaments, tendons, and the like. I often see cases in which otherwise fit weekend athletes come into my office with fatigue fractures of foot and leg bones because, although they still had plenty of bodily stamina left, some isolated but constantly used and reused bone did not. What happens in these instances is that while the rest of the body is standing up well to strenuous overall use in a sports activity, a particular bone that is the focus of that activity—again, usually an overworked foot or leg bone—cracks under the fatigue of constant pounding.

Of course, we should all remember that as we age, our bones become more brittle and more subject to injury than when we are younger. Thus, in addition to the elderly weekend athlete's precautions against overextending himself (his body's defense mechanisms will ensure that he doesn't in most instances), he should also take into account the increasing vulnerability of his bones when engaging in strenuous sports.

Aside from these general precautions, just about any recreational sport is open to any person who finds it to his liking. Even if you can only engage in your sport once a week, or once every ten days or two weeks, by all means do so. The infrequency of your activity may cause you aches, pains, and stiffness for a day or so afterward, but this is better than not giving your muscles, bones, and other body tissues any exercise at all. And there are easy ways by which you can prevent the post-participation aches and pains of infrequent, but at least regular, exercise. I shall explain these in a moment.

THE WEEKEND ATHLETE

You have no doubt gathered by now that by the term "weekend athlete" I am not referring to an individual who pursues his favorite athletic activity only on weekends. Of course, many of us are restricted to weekends throughout most of the year, but there are others, less numerous to be sure, who are able to engage in a sport two, three, and sometimes four times a week. For our purposes in this book, the more active participants qualify as weekend athletes, as do individuals who only participate in a sport sporadically. Both are basically amateur athletes who use their favorite sports as a form of recreation and exercise, and both are equally the victims of ailments that interfere with their enjoyment and ability to perform up to their usual skills.

NORMAL MISERIES OF
THE WEEKEND ATHLETE

Forgetting for the moment the chronic ailments that are the main subject of this book, the sporadic weekend athlete has it a bit tougher in the general aches-and-pains department than the more frequent recreational sports participant. This is because the frequent participant has the opportunity to keep his body —his bones, muscles, and connective tissues—in some semblance of condition vis-à-vis the sport he pursues, whereas the infrequent participant never gets his body in tune with his sport. Every individual, when first embarking on a sport, will feel muscle-and-joint aches and pains until the muscles he uses in that sport become conditioned to the stresses placed on them. The regular twice-a-week tennis player, the regular twice-a-week skier, the regular twice-a-week soccer player—all will be able to sustain their relevant muscles and body structures in a suitable state of tune so that normal post-participation aches and pains will occur minimally. The occasional, infrequent, or sporadic athletic participant, on the other hand—well, I'm sure you have all experienced the kind of Monday morning semi-paralysis I'm talking about, and that it needs no further description.

Aches, pains, and stiffness occur after unaccustomed physical activity for two reasons. The first is that in everyday—basically sedentary—life, your muscles, joints, tendons, ligaments, and other connective tissues are in a fairly lax and static state. This laxity becomes normal insofar as it is all that's required to meet your sedentary needs. Sudden participation in a sport after a considerable layoff, however—and the more physical the sport, the more acute are the effects—puts violent, abnormal stresses on the involved structural components. As muscles, ligaments, and tendons are repeatedly strained, contorted, and stretched the demand for blood to enable these areas to fulfill their functions increases markedly. The normal channels of blood supply, however, are not up to meeting the increased demand, and the situation becomes like trying to feed a 220-volt electric current through wires that are only capable of handling 110 volts. The wires heat up and possibly burn out, fuses blow, fire alarms sound!

Conditioning a body for a sport is mainly a process

of increasing the blood supply to the involved areas until the blood vessels can handle the demand, and increasing both the power and endurance of the muscles. Once this occurs, muscles and other parts can be repeatedly stressed without choking off blood-and-oxygen nourishment, and post-participation aches and pains no longer happen. One literally "conditions" the involved areas—that is, conditions the blood-supply process to respond to the increased demand by placing repeated stress on the involved areas until the supply is adequate to meet the needs of the muscles and other structures operating on a higher level of stress and strain than they are used to.

The weekend athlete who engages in a sport regularly every three or four days conditions himself mainly by the frequency of his participation—the muscles and other body parts become used to the stresses entailed by the sport and don't have a chance to become sedentary.

The true weekend athlete—the once-a-week sportsman—has it a little tougher. Because of the six- or seven-day interval between stresses and strains, his involved body parts tend to return to their normal, everyday laxity, and a mild form of Monday aches-and-pains is likely to result.

The infrequent sports participant has it toughest of all. If the interval between his or her participation in a sport is sufficient to allow body parts to return to their usual state, sports activities will just be one continual round of days-after aches, pains, stiffness, and sluggishness.

Such consequences, however—as I suggested earlier—can easily be avoided by keeping involved body parts in condition during the intervals between your sports activities. Many people believe that doing general setting-up exercises on a regular basis is all that's needed to prevent the normal aches and pains that result from once-a-week or less-frequent athletic activity. This is not necessarily true. Again, I do not want to minimize the virtues of regular setting-up exercises, and in no way do I wish to discourage you from engaging in them. They are certainly beneficial to your overall health and well-being. But for many sports, setting-up exercises alone are not sufficient for preventing the aches and stiffness that follow infrequent participation. Exercises are valuable in toning your overall musculature and in keeping you limber, but they usually do not reach or put great stress on the muscles and other tissues that come into most frequent play during a particular athletic activity.

For instance, simple setting-up exercises are not enough to condition all the specific muscles and tissues you use when you play three vigorous sets of tennis. They are not enough to condition all the muscles and tissues that receive great stress during a long afternoon of skiing. They are not enough even to condition all the muscles and tissues that are employed in so passive a game as golf.

If you do setting-up exercises regularly, I applaud you and recommend that you by all means continue them. Actually, for the non-athlete, they are very beneficial. But if you are a sporadic or weekend athlete and want to avoid pain-free Mondays when you do engage in a sport, I strongly suggest that you add to your repertoire of setting-up exercises one or two routines that are designed to work specifically on the structures of your body that receive the most stress during your favorite athletic activity. These exercises, done faith-

fully during the intervals between the times you engage in your favorite sport or sports, will not only
reduce the days of pain and stiffness you usually experience, they will also reduce the possibility of developing
a chronic or recurring ailment which could interfere
with your enjoyment and your ability to continue in the
sport.

Tennis elbow, for example, is an ailment that
plagues hundreds of thousands, maybe even millions of
amateur tennis players. I will get into this in considerably more detail in the chapter after next, but for now
I can say that among the key ingredients in the recipe
that produces tennis elbow are the muscles of the forearm—that is, unconditioned forearm muscles are often
the underlying cause of tennis elbow. If weekend tennis players were to do a daily exercise or two devoted
to conditioning and strengthening their forearm muscles, they would not only find less pain and stiffness in
their arms following several sets of tennis, they would
also be less likely to develop a case of tennis elbow.

ABNORMAL MISERIES OF
THE WEEKEND ATHLETE

The same holds true in any sport. Aches, pains, and
stiffness are the normal consequences of infrequent
athletic activity. But physical ailments—the ailments
that are the primary subject of this book—are another
consequence that is not so normal, even though their
frequency is definitely on the rise. With the increased
sports participation of recent years, they are in many
ways becoming the norm rather than the exception.

During each of the following chapters, when there

are specific exercises available that can help reduce your chances of suffering normal pain and stiffness after a particular athletic activity, I will outline one or two of the most effective of them. These exercises condition the specific structures of your body used in a sport and thereby reduce the normal aches and pains that usually follow. They also have the capacity to hasten the relief of the more serious sports-connected ailments and to prevent them from developing altogether.

Numerous among the patients I see are young men who painfully limp into my office on Monday mornings every fall with knees swollen to the size of Halloween pumpkins. Their medical history has usually been more or less the same. As high-school or college football players, they suffered debilitating knee injuries in which cartilages and/or ligaments were damaged. The result was that they invariably journeyed into adulthood with what are popularly known as "trick" knees. They retained their love for football, though, and indulged it by becoming regular weekend touch-football players.

On the particular Saturday or Sunday before their appearance in my office, they had been doing just that —playing in a game of touch football. As one who has played myself, I know how furious such games often become. Sure enough, these patients had taken a hit, or had pivoted the wrong way, or had done some acrobatic evasive maneuver during the previous weekend's game and suddenly found themselves on the ground with their knees as loose as a broken hinge, racked with pain and swelling like a soufflé.

Now the conditions with which they arrive at my office can no longer be classified as athletic ailments. They are out-and-out injuries that demand immediate and complex—often surgical—treatment to heal. But in many cases these severe knee injuries come about because their victims previously had an *ailment*—trick knee—which they had long neglected. Once a knee cartilage has been torn—the most common cause of trick knee—it can not repair itself because this cartilaginous tissue does not have any blood supply. Thus, once a person has suffered the original injury that caused trick knee to develop, unless the knee is surgically repaired, he or she is likely to remain with a trick knee for the rest of his or her life.

What occurs in the development of trick knee is that the original injury causes swelling all around the knee joint. After a while the swelling reduces, but the knee and the leg it is attached to remain relatively inactive for some time. This combination of factors causes the muscles which attach to and support the knee—especially the *quadriceps* muscles directly above the knee in the front of the thigh—to atrophy. These muscles shrink in size and lose much of their supportive strength. After the knee returns to more-or-less normal function, these muscles continue to exist in their withered and weakened state. Thus, an already compromised knee-joint is required to take on an even greater load than before it was injured because the supporting quadriceps muscles are never restored to their full supportive function. Because of this lack of stability, the knee is even more susceptible to reinjury. Such reinjury does not even require a traumatic blow; it can be triggered by something as seemingly harmless as a child hugging one's leg or a misstep off a curb.

The touch-football knee victims I see every fall invariably fit this profile. After their original knee injuries in high school or college, they neglected to restore their atrophied quadriceps muscles to full function.

Once their knees got "better," they found that they could get around pretty well without any further attention to them, and were troubled only occasionally when their knee "popped out of joint." Then came the fateful touch-football game, after which they ended up in my office.

Had they taken the trouble to do a specific and easy exercise to restore their withered quadriceps muscles the likelihood is that, although their knees would have remained "trick," they would never have had to come limping into my office with their swollen and still-further-damaged knees. Most such knee cases, when I ask them whether they have ever done quadriceps exercises, don't even know what I'm talking about—they have noticed for many years that one of their thighs is markedly thinner than the other, but have had no idea that this factor may well have contributed to their new injury.

By rebuilding the quadriceps muscles over the knee, an individual suffering from the ailment of trick knee returns much of the responsibility for the support of the knee to these muscles, where it belongs. Rebuilding the quadriceps beyond their former size and strength is further beneficial to the trick knee, and the chances of reinjury and further damage to the structures of the knee itself are all the more reduced. Once the quadriceps are rebuilt, they must then be maintained to keep them at ideal supportive strength. This can all be achieved through a simple leg-raising exercise. This exercise, which I will describe in more detail in the chapter on trick knee, will not only condition the muscles of your thigh, and thereby inhibit normal post-sports aches and pains in the area, it will also, in many cases, prevent the sports-related ailment of trick knee from turning into a serious knee injury. Of course, the avid athlete should also strengthen the other muscles of the leg and hip to provide his or her knee with additional support.

YOUR BODY, YOUR SPORT, YOUR MISERY

My original intention in this book was to divide it into chapters dealing with different sports and their specific ailments. However, many sports-connected ailments in the human body—and their concomitant miseries—cross the boundaries of different sports and affect participants in more than one activity. Thus, although such a format would have been convenient, it would have precluded discussing a number of ailments that are not associated with, or restricted to, one particular sport.

I am therefore dividing the book into chapters, each of which deals with a region of your body and the way its structures can develop ailments that are caused by particular sports, ailments which can interfere with your pleasurable participation in these sports and others.

I have already suggested that weekend athletic miseries fall into three categories—(1) normal aches and pains, (2) structural ailments, and (3) serious injuries—and have indicated how the first category can easily be overcome through specific conditioning exercises. Although certain miseries that fall under the category of "injuries" will be included in what follows, serious injuries are not our concern in this book except insofar as they can be prevented, as in the case of my example about trick knee. The treatment of sudden or serious injuries—fractured bones, joint dislocations, heart attacks, and the like—is purely a medical matter and best left to the hands and experience of the physician who treats you when and if you suffer such injuries.

That leaves us with what I have described as the frequent ailments associated with, or caused by, our athletic endeavors—tennis elbow, trick knee, bowler's thumb, golfer's hip, and so on.

There is an old saying that every human body is different. As a doctor who has seen and examined countless bodies over the years, I can attest to the truth of that axiom, but only in the aesthetic sense. I have seen thin bodies, fat bodies, short bodies, tall bodies, and just about every combination thereof. From the point of view of aesthetic proportions, no two bodies are the same.

But a body is more than the envelope in which a human being is contained—it is an incredibly complex and miraculously beautiful architectural structure that is made even more beautiful by the consistency of perfection with which it is reproduced almost every time a child is born. In this sense, then, no two bodies are different; every human body, with rare and freakish exceptions, is identically perfect and perfectly identical. Everything within the body, again with rare exception, is in its perfectly designed and functioning place, and each component operates in relationship to every other component with an identical and easy consistency that is mind-boggling when you stop to think about it.

Another way in which all bodies are the same is in their combination of durability and fragility, toughness and delicateness, solidity and flexibility. In the same way that the body is as sturdy as a truck engine, it is as brittle as a Swiss watch. And because of its delicacy, many things can go wrong with it.

The human body, despite its great flexibility, was not designed for use in athletic endeavors. As studies in genetics and evolution have shown us, the body makes gradual changes over the course of many generations to adapt itself to new environmental and cultural factors. But as far as I can tell it has not yet adapted itself to the golf swing, the screwball pitch, or the backhand smash.

Most of the sports-connected ailments that produce our athletic miseries involve the architectural components of our body's structure rather than its plumbing and heating systems. The bones, joints, muscles, tendons, ligaments, cartilage, and related tissues which make up the body's supportive musculo-skeletal system come most frequently under fire in athletic activities. It is these, either separately or in combination, which we'll be mostly considering in this book. Therefore, let us have a closer look at your body before we proceed further.

3

YOU AND YOUR BODY

I have learned through two decades of medical practice that many laymen are abysmally ignorant of the similarities and differences between the various parts of their musculo-skeletal anatomy, and that just as many are surprised when they discover there is more to the skeleton than just a bunch of bones. We've all heard the tune about the "headbone's connected to the neck bone, and the neck bone's connected to the shoulder bone . . ." etc. Many people's knowledge of their bodies doesn't go beyond that, which is unfortunate. It is unfortunate because a great deal of the misery involved in athletic misadventures would be avoided, I'm convinced, with a bit more knowledge about what one's body can and cannot effectively do within its particular limits.

25

The musculo-skeletal system of the body is made up not only of bones but also, as I have indicated, of joints, muscles, tendons, ligaments, cartilage, and other tissues which closely interact and interrelate to provide the body with its mobility and flexibility. In order to understand fully the nature and mechanics of the various sports ailments I am going to be discussing in the pages ahead—indeed, in order to understand the nature and mechanics of your own ailment—it is imperative that you know something about the nature and mechanics of the principal parts of your anatomy that come into play in these ailments.

YOUR BONES

You all know that bones are the basic girders of your skeletal frame. Many of you don't realize, though, that bones do quite a bit more than just serve as girders. Bone is the hardest substance in your body. It is composed of inorganic calcium salts and organic materials. Bones are living organisms, not the inert, lifeless objects that so many people believe them to be. They not only form the skeleton, they also have the functions of supporting various vital organs, producing blood cells, storing and releasing minerals to various parts of the body, and so on.

Bone is not the homogeneous object many believe it to be, either. It is composed of two components. One is the matrix, which is a protein substance upon which calcium salts are deposited to form the bone. The other is an intercellular substance which fills the microscopic spaces within the hardened calcium and acts as a sort of cement to hold the entire affair together.

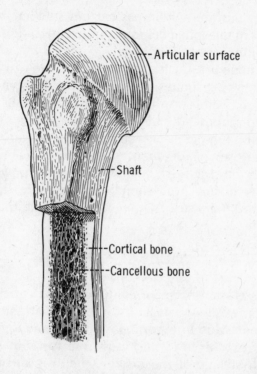

--Articular surface

--Shaft

--Cortical bone

--Cancellous bone

FIG. 1. *A cross section of the humerus, or upper-arm bone, showing the principal components and characteristics of the bone in your body.*

In addition to being formed of two components, bone also has two basic characteristics. We might call these "hard" and "soft." The deep interior or core of any bone is relatively soft when compared to the exterior, which is hard. This soft interior is known as the *cancellous* portion of the bone, while the hard exterior is known as the *cortical* portion. The proportion of hardness and softness varies among the bones of the body. The large structural bones tend to have a greater

degree of hardness, whereas certain smaller bones—
the bones in the spinal column, for instance—tend to be
on the softer side.

The bone in your body is as alive as the rest of you.
Portions of your bones are constantly dissolving and
new bone is being produced to replace it. It has been
calculated that every bone in an active person's body is
completely replaced over every seven-year period.
This is quite an achievement. Indeed, no other tissue in
your body has such excellent regenerative powers except for your skin. And when bones fracture, they heal
without leaving scars. Not even skin can do that.

YOUR MUSCLES

Here is another major component of the body that
too few people—especially weekend athletes—are
clear about. Muscle is composed of contractible fibers
that are responsive to impulses from the nerves. The
actual physiology of the nerve structures and muscle
reaction is quite complex and technical. It is sufficient
for our purposes to know that all the skeletal muscles
(those muscles which are attached to our bones and are
responsible for the motion of our skeletons) are controlled by our conscious thought processes. This is in
contrast to our internal organs, such as the heart, stomach, and intestines, which have muscles within them
but whose muscles are not controlled by voluntary impulse or conscious thought. You cannot will your heart
to slow down, or your stomach to stop growling when
you're hungry. But you certainly can will yourself to
pick up a ball, run a little faster or slower, or scratch
your ear.

Origins

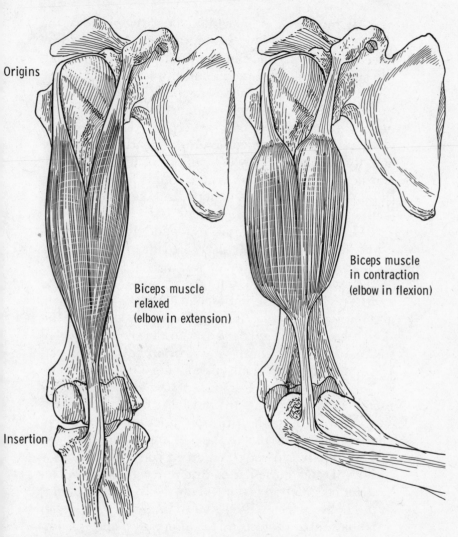

Biceps muscle
relaxed
(elbow in extension)

Biceps muscle
in contraction
(elbow in flexion)

Insertion

FIGS. 2 AND 3. *Two views of the major muscle of your upper arm—the biceps—while relaxed and contracted.*

All muscles are nourished on oxygen from the
body's circulating blood system and are controlled by
nerves which originate in the brain, descend through
the spinal cord, and branch out into the muscles. One
nerve may supply branches to many muscles, or one
muscle may have several branches from different
nerves. Therefore the contraction of a particular muscle may be partial or complete, depending upon the
activity of the nerves which supply it. It is this blood-
and-nerve supply system that accounts for such things
as muscle strength, muscle tone, muscle function, and
—muscle ache.

Muscles do not operate independently of one another. Muscles exist singularly and in groups. Within
each group muscles interact, and within specific areas
of the body various muscle groups interact with one
another. The body is composed of large, medium, small,
and miniscule muscles. Some lie near the surface of the
skin, others are buried deep within the skeleton, but all
function in an identical way. A brain cell is activated
and sends impulses along specific nerves that feed the
muscles. These impulses instantaneously stimulate a
muscle or group of muscles and cause them to contract.

Contraction is the primary function of muscles—
contraction is what moves the skeleton. Every time you
take a step, shift in your chair, turn your head, or chew
a piece of food, muscular contraction is the motive factor. But contraction is not the only role of the muscles
in the body. Muscles also serve to support the skeleton
and hold it together in proper alignment, and it is important that muscles be kept strong enough to fulfill
their supportive function. Many athletic ailments—as,
for instance, trick knee—are directly traceable to weak
muscle support around the affected joint areas. An-

other group of ailments often brought about by poor muscle support are back problems. The muscles of the back and abdominal areas are designed not only to provide movement and mobility but also to support the spine. When these muscles become too weak to properly do the job, the spine loses much of its support, its natural and correct curvature is altered, and disc and vertebrae problems result.

YOUR TENDONS

All parts and functions of the musculo-skeletal system are equally important, but each has its own special significance. The special significance of tendon is in its role of attaching muscle to bone. The tendons of your body are numerous and occur in many sizes, from very short and compact to very long and slender. Each tendon provides power and motion from the muscle out of which it grows to the bone to which it attaches.

Many people are perplexed by the various parts of the system and their different roles. They confuse tendons, ligaments, cartilages, and other components, and will often mistakenly describe a cartilage problem as a ligament or tendon problem, and vice versa. So let me repeat what tendons do: they connect or attach the muscles of your body to its bones. It is in this function that tendons become the source of so much misery in athletic endeavors, for when a weak or unconditioned muscle is overextended, it can stretch one or more of its bone attachments (tendons) or even cause them to separate partially from the bone, thus causing inflammation and pain.

Tendons are dense, tough, and relatively inflexible.

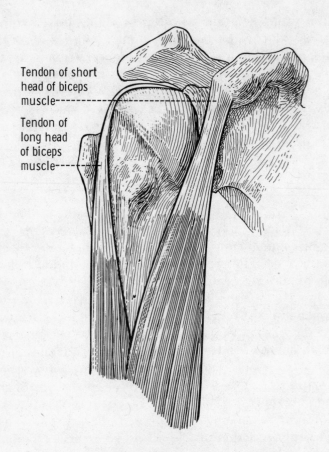

Tendon of short
head of biceps
muscle----------

Tendon of
long head
of biceps
muscle----

FIG. 4.   *A view of two of the many tendons of your*
shoulder, showing how tendons attach muscle to
bone.

They are neither muscle nor bone, but a stiff cord or
band of fibrous tissue. Although the word "tendon" derives from the Latin verb for "to stretch," its name is
misleading because tendons do not have an unlimited
stretch capacity; indeed, most ailments involving ten-

dons occur when they are abnormally stretched. Tennis elbow is probably the most frequent manifestation of a tendon's inability to bear much stretching.

YOUR LIGAMENTS

Any sports fan knows the importance of ligaments. "Joe Namath has torn ligaments in both knees and cannot run." "Jean-Claude Killy almost tore the ligaments in his right ankle during the slalom." "Reggie Jackson ruptured some ligaments in his back and will miss the World Series." Ligaments are indeed important. But how many of you know what they are and what they do?

The first thing we should be clear about is that ligaments, like tendons, are dense, stiff, very strong bands of fibrous tissue. The major difference between the two is in their functions. Whereas tendons attach muscle to bone, ligaments *attach one bone to another.* Ligaments go from one bone to the next and hold them together in their proper relationships. They are more flexible than tendons, so that a certain amount of motion can occur at their connecting joints, but at the same time they have, again like tendons, a low amount of elasticity. Thus they can be stretched only to a limited degree before they rupture or "tear."

Once a ligament has been torn, it does not repair itself. When it is either partially or completely torn, it relaxes the normal tension holding a joint's parts in their proper relationship, and the joint loosens. Such looseness can then provoke all sorts of further complications, such as instability (e.g., trick knee), arthritis, and so on. It can also have a deleterious effect on nearby

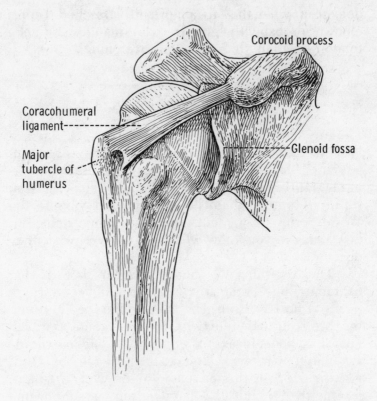

FIG. 5. *A view of one of the many ligaments of your shoulder, showing how ligaments attach bone to bone.*

areas of the body. A ligament can only be repaired surgically—that is, through a procedure of removing the section of ligament which is torn or ruptured, then inserting other tissue to replace it.

Ligaments are numerous throughout the body. Not only do they join every bone to every other bone, they also figure importantly in every articulating joint.

The principal function of ligaments in joints is to provide a checkrein effect so that joints cannot overextend in an unnatural direction and tear or pull apart all the muscles and other structures surrounding them. Probably the most frequently noticed ligaments are those in the knee, but ligaments have equally vital functions throughout the body. The ligaments of the spine, for instance, hold the spinal column in its proper alignment. Each of the twenty-four vertebrae in your back, and corresponding discs, represents a joint; thus you have twenty-four small articulating joints in your spine. The various spinal ligaments keep these joints connected and in line, and prevent the spine from overextending under normal conditions.

YOUR CARTILAGES

I include cartilages at this point in our brief musculo-skeletal survey because, even though they do not figure as importantly as ligaments and tendons in overall body function, they are probably the most misunderstood of the three when it comes to sports-connected ailments, especially those having to do with the knee. We hear a great deal about people suffering "torn cartilages" when what is really meant is that they have suffered torn ligaments or ruptured tendons.

First of all, the word cartilage comes from the Latin word for "gristle," and that's precisely what cartilage is—a tough, dense, rubbery tissue that can only be called gristle. In the human body cartilage exists in two forms, and this is where the confusion arises. In the first and more common form, it exists as a translucent, membranous covering on the ends of bones where they rub against each other at the joints. It secretes a lubricating fluid and serves as one of several lubricating mechanisms in the body's joints.

But it is not in this form that cartilage comes into play in relation to sports ailments. Cartilage also exists in the form of flat, rubbery, crescent-shaped discs within the knee joint.* Their function is to help ease the articulation of the joint surfaces. Although they are often called the "cartilages" of the knee, their proper name in medical terminology is "meniscus" in the singular and "menisci" in the plural (from the Greek word *meniskos*, which means "crescent"). No matter what we call them, they are capable of being fragmented or ripped away from their connections in the knee during a sudden, abnormal motion of the knee. When this occurs, the fragment then floats loose in the knee and usually lodges between the two articulating surfaces, causing friction, inflammation, pain, and interference with joint motion.

YOUR JOINTS

Here we arrive at the most important components of your body—important insofar as they permit you to engage in your favorite sports. Without joints, we would all move about quite a bit differently than we do, and our sports and games would probably look like they belonged on another planet. Our joints are the central focus of all that has gone before in the form of the bones, muscles, tendons, and ligaments that make up

---

*It might also be noted that the famous discs of the spine are capsules, the upper and lower walls of which are made of cartilage tissue.

our musculo-skeletal system, and they are what give us our bodily mobility and flexibility. They are also the most frequent site of our sports-associated miseries.

The three most common types of joints in the body are: the *ball-and-socket* (hip, shoulder); the *hinge* (knee, elbow); and the *modified-hinge,* often called a "saddle joint" (ankle, thumb). The ball-and-socket joints are the largest and, anatomically, the least complicated. They allow for the greatest range of motion, and except for dislocations (which usually result from sudden injuries) and inflammations of their *bursa,* little goes wrong with them under ordinary athletic conditions. Of course, inflammations of the bursa—flat, membranous sacs which protect the movement of the joints from interference by other tissues—can be very painful ailments indeed. They go under the name of *bursitis* and occur most frequently in the ball-and-socket joints —the hip and the shoulder.

The hinge joints are smaller structures but quite a bit more complicated than the ball-and-socket joints; thus they are subject to a greater variety of ailments. The range of motion they permit is limited. For instance, the knee and elbow joints are limited to forward-backward articulation only, with the backward articulation (flexion) capable of full range and the forward articulation (extension) capable of half the range. If you hold your arm straight out in front of you with your elbow stationary, you should be able to bend it back so that your hand touches your shoulder; this is the *full-flexion* capability of your elbow. Now extend your arm again and you will find that it returns to the straight position, but no further. This is the elbow's *maximum extension* capability. If your arm were to go beyond its normal straightness, and the crook of your elbow were to bend backward, it would mean that something was wrong with your elbow joint. Women's elbows are naturally more supple, however, and can normally hyperextend five-to-ten degrees.

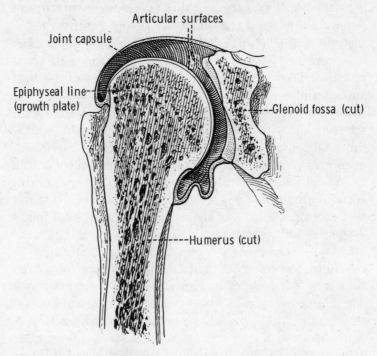

FIG. 6.　*A view of your shoulder joint, showing the ball-and-socket effect, the articular surfaces, and the joint's capsule.*

Try the same thing with your leg. Standing with your legs straight, flex one knee and raise your heel as high as you can behind you (if you are really agile you should be able to touch your heel to your buttocks). Then return it to its straight position and notice how it cannot extend *beyond* the straight. If it does, there is again something probably wrong with your knee joint.

These little exercises illustrate the full-flexion and extension capabilities of your hinge joints. What energizes the movement of these joints is, of course, as with all your joints, your muscle-nerve complex. But the mechanics of joint function itself depends on the bones, ligaments, tendons, and other supporting and articulating components within the joints. These components regulate and harmonize the movements of the joints. They also limit those motions the joints are not designed to make and which would be injurious if they were made.

I come to a point now when I would like to emphasize the motions of *flexion* and *extension,* for these are the basic functions of the muscles that come into play in a great variety of athletic movements and maneuvers, and are also the two primary forms of joint movement.

Two of the major types of muscles we have throughout our bodies are what are known as *flexor* and *extensor* muscles. Our flexor muscles work in conjunction with our joints to produce flexion. Our extensor muscles work to produce extension. Hold one of your arms out again, for example. Now, flex your elbow—that is, bend it so that your hand comes back to touch your shoulder. As you do so place the fingers of your free hand on the biceps surface—the front portion—of your upper arm and feel how the biceps muscles contract. Then, as you extend your elbow, returning your arm to the straight position, place your fingers on the triceps surface—the rear portion—of your upper arm and feel how the triceps muscles contract when your arm reaches its straight and fully extended position.

This exercise illustrates how all the muscles in your body work when you make a joint movement—even down to the tiniest joints in your fingers and toes. Your muscles *always contract,* but some contract for the purposes of flexion—these are the flexor muscles—and some for the purposes of extension—the extensor muscles. I shall discuss the flexor and extensor muscles in quite a bit of detail in the chapters ahead, so it is important that you have a clear preliminary picture of their functions and how they work.

There are two other muscle types that work in conjunction with joint motion, and of these you should also be aware. They are the *abductor* and *adductor* muscles. These function mainly in concert with the ball-and-socket joints—the hips and shoulders. *Abduction,* in anatomical terms, means to draw away from the midline of the body. The act of raising your arm away from your side or swinging your hips laterally or spreading your legs is an *abductive* movement. The *abductor* muscles of your shoulder or hip lie along the outer aspects of these joints and are the principal muscles that enable the joints to perform these movements.

Adduction (note the difference between "ab" and "ad") means just the opposite of abduction: it means to draw toward the midline of the body. The act of lowering your arm or pressing and holding your legs together is an act of *adduction.* The adductor muscles of your hip or shoulder are located interiorly to these joints and are somewhat offset from them. Your shoulder's adductor muscles, for instance, are located below—forward and behind—the shoulder joints. Your hip's adductor muscles are located in your groin; they enable you to pull your legs together and also provide support and stability in your pelvic region.

These general muscle groups are each made up of many different, individual muscles—some deep, others near the skin's surface. For instance, the hip adductors comprise five major muscles plus a series of smaller ones, all of which interrelate and interact every time you perform an adduction movement. One of the hip adductors is known as the *gracilis* muscle (all muscles in the body are known by Latin names). This gracefully named muscle, because it holds the legs together, has often been referred to as the guardian of virginity—at least in days of yore!

The hip and shoulder joints also have their own flexor and extensor muscles, and it is the combination of all these, along with the ball-and-socket geometry of the joints themselves, that permits such a complete range of motion in the hips and shoulders—as opposed to the hinge joints of the body, whose motion is restricted to flexion and extension.

The third type of joint in your body is the *modified-hinge*, or *saddle*, joint, of which the ankle is the most readily visible example. The ankle is the joint that connects the foot to the leg. It is called a "saddle" joint because the major bone of the joint—the *talus*, or ankle bone—is shaped like an inverted saddle. But the movement at the joint—where the lower end of the leg bone, or tibia, meets the top of the ankle bone—is limited, as is the movement of the elbow or the knee, to flexion and extension. The ankle joint is held together by the usual assortment of tendons, ligaments, and muscles, and of course it is just as subject to injuries and ailments involving these components as are other joints. I will get into the construction of the various joints of the body in more detail further on when I explain their specific ailments.

YOUR CIRCULATORY SYSTEM

The important thing to remember here is that every portion of your body is kept alive by your blood-supply, or circulatory, system. In that sense, of course, your circulatory system is the most vital component in your musculo-skeletal structure. You can get along without certain joints, muscles, tendons, bones, what-have-you, but without your circulatory system you would soon pass into another world—one which, as far as I know, doesn't feature sports.

Your circulatory system is made up of heart, lungs, arteries, veins, and capillaries of progressively diminishing size that reach into the farthest and deepest recesses of your body to nourish them with blood. The arteries in our bodies carry fresh oxygenated blood from our hearts to all our body cells, and without the oxygen provided by the blood, none of these cells could survive. Our brain cells are the most susceptible to decreased oxygen supply and will die after only four minutes of oxygen deprivation. Muscles, bones, and associated tissues and cells, on the other hand, can last an hour or more without oxygen.

Once fresh blood is delivered by our arteries and is absorbed by our cells and tissues, it becomes, so to speak, used blood. The veins in our bodies pick up the used blood, which now has a high carbon dioxide content, and return it, along their various byways, to the heart, which then recycles it through our lungs to rid it of its carbon dioxide wastes and infuse it with fresh oxygen (if such is available in these days of increasing air pollution).

That, in a nutshell, is our circulatory system. But

like everything else, it can go wrong and cause a variety of problems throughout our bodies. Two fundamental things that can go wrong with our circulatory system are: (1) either the arteries are for some reason unable to deliver fresh blood in the required amounts to the intended destinations; or (2) the veins are for some reason unable to return the used blood to the factory—the heart—for recycling.

Let us assume that the heart is not the culprit in the breakdown of the system, although it often is. If the heart is working normally as an efficient pump, clean, fresh blood will be sent out through the arteries. But if there is an obstruction in one or more of the arteries— a clot or *embolus*—the blood will not be able to get through. Or if the clot is partial, only an insufficient flow of blood is possible. Thus, a partial or complete arterial embolism is one possible cause of a breakdown in the circulatory system.

Another results from a narrowing of the arterial tubes, as happens in *arteriosclerosis*, or hardening of the arteries. Again, the proper flow of blood is diminished, and the vital parts of the body supplied by the affected artery are deprived of the blood nourishment they require.

When the cells of muscle and other body tissues are suddenly and completely deprived of blood, they will die after an hour or two. If the supply of blood is diminished but is still sufficient to keep the cells and tissues alive, they will continue to live but will have little or no tolerance for activity. Activity, therefore—the normal activity of supporting a particular body structure, but even more so the intense activity of certain sports—will produce fatigue, debility, pain, and any number of

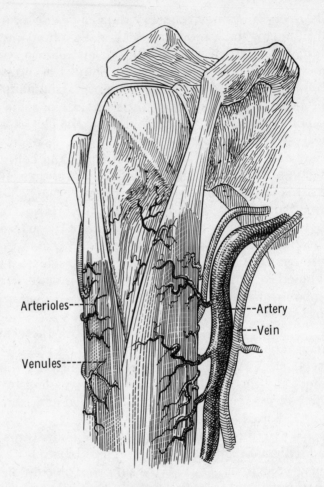

Arterioles

Artery

Vein

Venules

FIG. 7. *A view of how the blood-supply system feeds the tissues of the upper arm.*

other unpleasant and enjoyment-reducing symptoms. An insufficient blood supply can also cause the affected parts of the body to be more readily injured, or chronically diseased.

Breakdowns in the veins are generally less serious than arterial obstructions, but can also produce severe fatigue and pain. *Varicose veins* are often the source of leg pain. By itself, such a condition can interfere with one's enjoyable participation in sports activities. When the pain radiates upward through the lower parts of the torso it can make such activities positively agonizing. *Thrombophlebitis,* or inflammations of the veins, is another villain. When the veins become inflamed, they slowdown the return of used blood to the heart. As the blood backs up it begins to stagnate. Clots form, which then may break off and be carried to the heart and lungs, causing damage there.

This short description of the functions of the circulatory system is not meant to teach you all you have to know about it, it is merely designed to make you aware of the vitally important role the system plays, not only in your normal activities but in your athletic endeavors as well. Most people fail to take into account their blood-supply system when thinking about their particular athletic ailments, yet an adequate and properly composed blood supply is central to the ailment-free enjoyment of sports, not to mention life itself.

Another item people fail to take into account are their lungs. I very seldom encounter a patient who is actively aware of the correlation between his or her circulatory system and lungs. We've already seen how diminished blood supply, or a diminution in the proper levels of oxygen in the blood, can cause the fatiguing and weakening of body cells and tissues. Blocked or narrowed arteries are only one way in which body parts can be deprived of normal blood nourishment. Another occurs when used blood recycled by the heart cannot obtain the proper amounts of oxygen from the lungs.

Now, I am sure all of you who smoke have grown exceedingly tired of the admonishments you receive from family, concerned friends, even doctors, so I'm not going to add to the clamor by telling you that every cigarette you light is another nail in your coffin. Yet you should understand that aside from being eminently unhealthful under normal circumstances, smoking also severely restricts any gains you receive through the exercise associated with your athletic activities. It also increases your chances of developing a sports-connected ailment and reduces your chances of getting rid of it. How?

Most people believe that the only misery smoking produces in athletic activities is short-windedness, and they are willing to sacrifice their reduced wind in exchange for the pleasure of smoking. But short-windedness is more than just an annoying by-product of smoking; it is also a symptom of the lungs' inability to provide normal and sufficient levels of oxygen to the blood-supply system. And I have noted what occurs in the body when blood supply or its oxygen content is reduced: body parts—their cells and tissues—are forced to function at diminished efficiency and reduced tolerance. They not only fatigue more readily, they also fail to return to normal function as quickly as when they have an adequate blood and oxygen supply. What functions they *are* capable of carrying out are done under the increased threat of further debility or injury.

For the individual with a specific arterial problem, the deleterious effect of reduced blood supply or diminished blood content will usually pertain to only one region of the body. For the smoker, on the other hand, the effects occur throughout his entire body; every region, every cell, every tissue receives diminished oxygen supply.

I shall be talking more about blood supply and its role in athletic miseries as we go along, but it is important that you have an overview of the general picture now so that you can appreciate the importance of a healthy circulatory system to the pursuit of athletic pleasure. Smoking is unhealthy not only because it *can* cause lung cancer but also because it *will* cause circulatory inefficiency.

YOUR NERVOUS SYSTEM

With the nervous system we come to the final important component of your musculo-skeletal structure. It is also probably the least understood of all the vital systems within the body.

Most people correctly understand that their nerves are what actually account for pain, but they have very little idea of how the pain-nerve relationship works. One of the more common misconceptions I find people holding is the notion that nerves are isolated points in the body and that if one is "hit" it will create pain.

This, of course, is nonsense. Nerves are not isolated points, but a complex network of lines which, like your blood vessels, run throughout your body and reach into its every area. Indeed, your nervous system can be compared directly to your circulatory system. Just as your circulatory system is controlled and operated by one organ—the heart—so too is the nervous system controlled by the brain. And just as your circulatory system consists of hollow vessels that carry blood from your heart and then return it, so too does your nervous system consist of vessels—although not hollow—that carry impulses both to and from your brain.

It has become fashionable these days to compare

the brain to a computer, as if that makes it easier for us to understand what the brain is. Perhaps it does make it easier—for the computer expert. But I'm not a computer expert. Nor, I expect, are most of you.

Basically, your brain is the master control system of the entire organism that is your body. It controls the vast network of what we call nerves—the electric wires of our system—which, in turn, control and affect every portion of your body.

A nerve is a cordlike or filamentous band of tissue composed essentially of fibers capable of conducting the electric impulses produced by the brain. Thousands of these bands or cords, large and small, are to be found in the body. The larger of them emanate from centers in the brain; they then travel through the spinal cord and, by means of hundreds of branches and sub-branches of all lengths and thicknesses, reach into every part of the body. Through its branches and sub-branches, the nervous system coordinates and regulates the excitation of muscles, organs, and glands, and directly conditions all behavior and activity.

In man, the nervous system has two major components: the *somatic* system and *autonomic* system. The somatic system is the combination of brain and spinal-cord nerves which governs our voluntary actions, motions, and sensory feelings. The autonomic system is part of the peripheral system that governs our involuntary actions, motions, and feelings, such as those pertaining to circulation, digestion, and the like. Both systems are interrelated and are part of the central nervous system, but for our purposes here we are more concerned with the somatic system, mainly because it is directly involved in our athletic activities and the ailments and miseries that derive therefrom.

Our somatic nervous system carries commands from our brain to our muscles and enables the muscles to contract, thereby producing the movements we desire to make. You will recall that within your blood-supply system there are two primary kinds of carriers: arteries and veins. Similarly, in your nervous system there are two basic kinds of nerves: the *sensory nerves,* often called "receptors," and the *motor nerves,* often called "effectors." The sensory, or receptor, nerves receive stimuli from within or without the body and instantaneously transmit the sensations received back to the brain center. There the sensations are interpreted, again instantaneously, and acted upon by the appropriate stimulation of the motor, or effector, nerves. Each body part has a sensory and motor nerve which connects to the brain through the complex network of nerve branches and subbranches.

A simple example of how the entire two-way nerve system works is when you accidentally touch your finger to a hot stove. The receptor nerve endings in your finger are immediately stimulated (your nerves have hot-and-cold sensory endings, as well as endings for countless other sensations), and an electrical charge is flashed through your nerve network to your brain. The brain receives the informational impulses and refers them to an "action center." The action center instantaneously sends an impulse down along the appropriate effector, or motor pathway, that reaches into your finger and controls the muscles associated with the finger and its motor-nerve endings. Suddenly, the finger is jerked away from the stove. The entire sequence occurs a hundred times faster than the blink of an eye. We have all actually experienced it, or something like it, countless times in our lives.

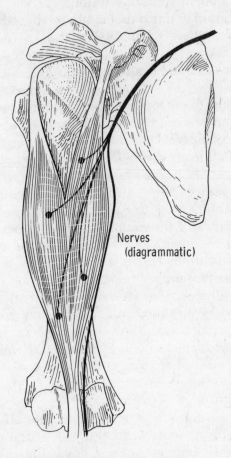

Nerves
(diagrammatic)

FIG. 8.   *The nerve of the upper-arm muscles.*

It all sounds very simple, doesn't it? In fact, the
whole process of action-reaction is considerably more
complicated than I have described. All of our thousands
of nerve cells and their branches have a maze of inter-
connecting links, so that very few isolated activities

occur. Often we receive stimuli through one area of our body and react in another. It is this capability that enables us to engage in hundreds of different activities, including sports.

For instance, when we are on the tennis court and see the ball speeding across the net toward us, a variety of receptor nerves are activated, including those connected to our eyes. Our visual sensations are instantaneously processed through the memory storehouse of our brains, referred to its action center, and translated through the appropriate motor-nerve pathways to various parts of our bodies. Thus we run to meet the ball, swing our racket, follow through, and so on. The process is a continuing one—an infinite number of instantaneous action-reaction-action moments—and is illustrative of how complex and reflexive most of our learned activities are.

But our nervous system is not only the fundamental means by which we can accomplish all the wonderful things we do. It is also the source of pain. Moreover, when nerves are damaged, it can be the source of physical weakness or disability as well. These are facts that exemplify my earlier contention that there can be no pleasure in life without pain, and vice versa. Life is indeed a process of contrasts and contradictions.

YOUR PAIN

Just as through our nervous systems we are capable of delighting in a spectrum of beautiful colors, of tasting delicious foods, of experiencing the pleasurable warmth of a loved one's caresses, of stroking a golf ball far and true, so too are we capable of feeling the emo-

tional grief of bad news and the physical pain of an
inflamed muscle or joint. Although we owe to our
nerves the sensations of pleasure we enjoy, to them also
do we owe the pain we endure.

Your body is part of nature, and it exists in a balance of all sorts of opposing and contrasting forces—just
as nature itself does. When your body is in a normal
state of health, you experience neither extraordinary
pleasure nor extraordinary pain from it. When everything is working properly, there is no reason why you
should have pleasurable sensations in your body, or
painful ones. The only pleasure you should receive is a
spiritual one, the kind that derives from knowing that
you have no pain.

But let something go wrong, let the balance get
tipped, and pain is your reward. Not only the spiritual
pain that comes from worry or anxiety about your condition, but real live pain—the kind that hurts a specific
part of your body. Body pain comes in a variety of
shapes, sizes and intensities. These all depend on a
number of things: the nature of your disorder, the site
at which the disorder occurs, and the cause. Notwithstanding these factors, however, the real source of the
pain you feel, whether mild or excruciating, are your
sensory nerves and the motor-nerve reactions they produce. Note that I said they are the source, not the cause,
of your pain.

Your nervous system operates throughout your
body in exactly the same way it functions in your
fingers. Remember the "hot stove" example I used
before? Well, your entire body is full of hot stove pos-
sibilities.

As you have learned, your body is one vast, complex system of sensory and motor nerves hooked into

your main nervous system. You possess big nerves, medium-sized nerves, small nerves, tiny nerves, miniscule nerves, thousands of them, all running to and from hundreds of specific sites in your body, and infiltrating every last fiber, tissue, and cell. When you touch your finger to a hot stove, the cluster of sensory nerve endings flashes the message to your brain, which in turn flashes back the command through your body's effector nerve circuit that enables you to withdraw your finger from the stove in a reflexive reaction designed to *relieve* the pain. All in less than a twinkling.

The entire process of other pains in the body works in the same way—with one exception. First, you have a cause; but instead of it being a hot stove, it's a torn muscle, an overstretched tendon, a ruptured ligament, a hyperextended joint, a chipped and inflamed bone, or any of dozens of other possible imbalances. The cause —whatever it might be—instantly alerts the sensory nerve fibers feeding the particular part of your body that is affected. These sensory nerves, which are tied into your main nerve cables, flash the message to your brain. The brain pulls the alarm, so to speak, and lights start blinking in its action center, bells start clanging, sirens start wailing—Pain! Now your effector nerves mobilize as your brain shoots messages back to the affected site.

But in this case you cannot lift the affected part off the stove. If you were to have voluntarily kept your finger on the stove in our earlier example, your pain would have increased and you would have suffered a severe burn, with all of its further and even more painful consequences. However, you *were* able to withdraw it, and did so in a reflexive neurological reaction. The precipitating cause of the pain was outside your body,

the pain itself was on a surface of your body, and your
neurological reactions relieved the pain.

But once pain has been precipitated within your
body by some cause outside it—by the faulty swinging
of a racket, for instance, or the incorrect use of your
palm in a handball game—the *precipitating cause* is no
longer a factor. It is the *underlying cause* of pain—the
relationship between the injured or damaged body part
and your nervous system—that becomes your concern.
And there is no way you can remove or withdraw, as in
my finger-stove illustration, your affected body part
from the *underlying cause.*

The underlying cause of your pain is imprisoned
within your body. The neurological reflex to "withdraw" the affected body part from the source of its pain
is compromised; there is no place to withdraw to. What
occurs, then, is that your effector, or motor, nerves,
trying to help your afflicted body part recoil from the
source of its pain, are stymied. Their effort, however,
produces spasm and further pain—especially when the
afflicted part is moved or additionally stressed.

Although I have oversimplified it, this is the basic
nature and mechanics of body pain. There are countless
variations on this theme, but they all add up to the same
thing—anything from mild discomfort to exquisite
agony, depending upon the nature, site, and causes of
the ailment, and also upon dozens of other factors including time, severity, and the general condition of
your body.

So much, then, for our general study of the body
and the way in which our athletic ailments and their
accompanying miseries can arise. I am sure you are
now anxious to press on into specifics. In the chapters
immediately following I'll take you on the journey

through the thick forest of athletic ailments—their causes, symptoms, treatments, and the preventive measures you can take to avoid, control, or overcome them. I am certain that at some point along the way we'll come to your particular problem. It's my hope that once you recognize it and gain a better understanding of it, you'll then be ready, willing, and able to deal with it the way it should be dealt with—all for the purpose of increasing your enjoyment of your favorite sports.

4

YOUR ELBOW MISERIES —TENNIS ANYONE?

TENNIS ELBOW

A handshake becomes an ordeal. Turning a doorknob sends arrows of searing pain through your forearm. Lifting a cup of tea or brushing your teeth is an agonizing experience. And swinging a racket at a tennis ball—especially if the ball hits off center—causes a sensation that some tennis players compare with being struck on the elbow with a hot poker or with the full force of a sledgehammer.

These are all symptoms of an ailment that has long been familiar to doctors and athletes but is now becoming epidemic in America: "Tennis Elbow." With an estimated 11 million Americans playing tennis for fun and exercise, and an additional half-million taking up the game each year, tennis elbow has become easily the most frequent and common source of athletic misery.

Javelin throwers, football and baseball players, golfers, and even violinists often suffer identical symptoms—indeed, anyone who uses his arm to any great extent in a sport or vocation is susceptible to the disorder.

THE SOURCES OF TENNIS ELBOW

My coauthor, Thomas Kiernan, developed a case of tennis elbow a few years ago, even though he never played tennis. It made his everyday life pretty miserable and acutely interfered with his enjoyment of the sports he did play, such as golf and touch football (he couldn't throw a football more than ten yards, a pretty dismal prospect for a former quarterback). After asking him a few questions when he came to my office looking for help, I was able to determine the *precipitating cause* of his ailment: he had spent the previous few weeks chopping down trees with an ax while clearing a field on an old farm he shared with his family. He was not a woodsman by vocation, in fact he had never used an ax before. It was obvious that the unaccustomed strain on his elbow-forearm complex, which resulted from the repeated jarring of the ax, was at the root of his problem.

This is just one illustration of how tennis elbow can come about. It also illustrates the fundamental mechanics surrounding the development of the condition—repeated traumatic stress on the unconditioned elbow-forearm complex through unnatural arm motions at

moments of impact. Yet despite the fact that tennis
elbow can happen to anyone, it is because of the mushrooming popularity of tennis that doctors' waiting
rooms are filling up at an unprecedented rate with victims of the ailment. And it is because it occurs more
frequently in tennis players than in anyone else that it
gets its popular name—although in medical terminology it is known as *"lateral epicondylitis."*

You would do well to note here, since I will occasionally be using general medical terms throughout the
book, that in medicine "lateral" refers to the outer portions of any given body part and "medial" refers to the
inner portions. Similarly, "posterior" refers to the rear
portions, and "anterior" refers to the front portions. It
would also be well to note, if you're not already aware
of it, that any medical term that has the suffix "itis"
attached to it means an infection and/or inflammation
of the body part described by that term (appendicitis,
for example, means an infection and inflammation of
the appendix).

SOME ELBOW ANATOMY

Lateral epicondylitis, the medical name for tennis
elbow, means, then, that the outer epicondyle of the
elbow is inflamed.* But what, you ask, is an epicondyle?
In order to understand this better—indeed, in order to
understand the entire structure of the elbow-forearm
complex—we should take a more detailed look at the
region.

---

*There is also an elbow condition we doctors call *medial epicondylitis,*
which is more popularly known as "thrower's elbow." It involves the inner
aspects of the elbow, whereas lateral epicondylitis, or tennis elbow, involves
the outer aspects. I shall discuss thrower's elbow further on in this chapter.

It goes without saying that the elbow is one of the most important joints in the body, and is especially important to anyone who enjoys sports activities in which the arm plays a central role (there are, of course, very few sports in which the arm doesn't play a central, or at least supporting, role). It also goes without saying that until something goes wrong with it, we tend to take our elbow very much for granted.

As I have already indicated, the elbow is one of the hinge joints of the body: it is capable of moving only in one plane, like a hinge. It is a joint that comprises the bone of the upper arm (the *humerus*) and the two long bones of the lower arm (the *radius,* which extends along the outer aspect of the forearm, and the *ulna,* which extends along the inner aspect).

The humerus, which is the long bone of the upper arm connecting the elbow to the shoulder, is roughly circular for most of its length. However, it widens and flattens at its lower, or elbow, terminus and forms into two rounded knobs—one on the inner side and one on the outer side of the end of the bone. These knobs are called the *trochlea* and the *capitulum* and are the upper articulating surfaces of the elbow joint. (By the "articulating surfaces" of any joint I mean the end portions of two adjoining bones that move against one another when motion occurs in that joint.)

Behind the two knobs forming the lower end of the humerus is a depression, or notch, called the *olecranon notch.* This notch helps to prevent the elbow from extending beyond its capability when the arm is held straight.

The radius and ulna—the two bones of the forearm —connect the elbow to the wrist. They are both equal in length, but the radius—the outer bone of the forearm—is roughly twice the diameter of the ulna. The

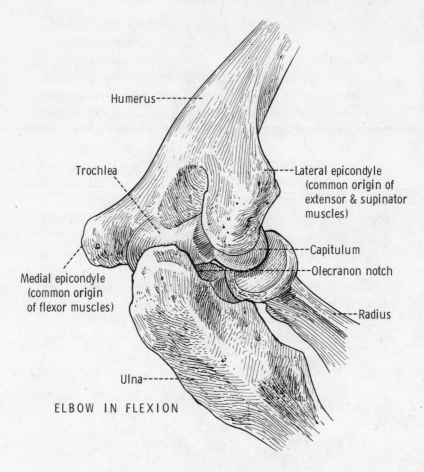

FIG. 9. *The skeletal components of your elbow. Note the lateral epicondyle; then the medial epicondyle.*

upper end of the radius is rounded and contains a small concave depression at its tip into which fits the outer rounded knob at the lower end of the humerus—the capitulum. The ulna has a deep cup at its upper end, and into it fits the inner rounded knob at the lower end of the humerus—the trochlea. In addition, a portion of the ulna projects beyond this notch like a finger; the projection, called the *olecranon process*, fits into the olecranon notch behind the two knobs at the lower end of the humerus. This projection and its corresponding notch provide the elbow with its locking action, preventing it from overextension.

This, essentially, is the bony construction of the elbow joint. The two knobs at the end of the humerus (the upper arm bone) articulate with the tips of the radius and ulna of the forearm. In addition, a secondary bone articulation takes place between the olecranon process and the olecranon notch at the rear of the joint. You can see, then, that the mechanics of motion in the elbow joint is a fairly simple matter. But this is not all there is to it.

Many people tend to believe that most elbow problems arise out of breakdowns in the bone-to-bone action of the elbow joint. Such, however, is not the case. Of course, such things as elbow arthritis can occur in the conjunction of bones in the elbow, but these are not very frequent here, and when they do occur they are not usually sports-related ailments. The sports-related ailments such as tennis elbow are much more common disorders of this joint, and they occur precisely because there is much more to elbow motion than simply the articulation of the lower- and upper-arm bones where they meet in the joint. And this brings us to the *epicondyles*, after which tennis elbow (and thrower's elbow) gets its medical name.

THE LATERAL AND MEDIAL EPICONDYLES

You will recall from the last chapter that the joints of the body consist of more than just two or more bones coming together. Every joint has ligaments and other components that hold it together, support it, lubricate it and otherwise aid in its articulation. Moreover, except by gravity, no joint can move on its own; it requires a wide variety of muscles surrounding it, nourished by blood supply and sensitized by nerve input, to move it. These muscles must, of course, be attached to the joint in various ways to enable it to move in accordance with its anatomical design.

You will also recall from the last chapter that tendons are the parts in your body whose specific function it is to attach the appropriate muscles in your body to your bones. It is in this function—the attachment of muscle to bone in your elbow joint—that the *underlying cause* of the miseries of tennis elbow is to be found. So, although I want to keep the explanations in this book as straightforward and nontechnical as possible, we must go beyond our understanding of the simple bone-to-bone mechanics of elbow articulation and understand the muscle-to-bone relationship—how it functions and how it can cause the trouble that results in tennis elbow.

To achieve this understanding, we must first return our attention to the lower end of the humerus (the bone of the upper arm). The primary function of the lower end of the humerus is to articulate, by means of its twin terminus knobs and its posterior notch, with the upper ends of the radius and ulna and with the posterior knob of the ulna. But the lower end of the humerus has another function which in its own way is just as important, and that is to serve as the principal site of attachment for the various muscles that come into play in elbow movement. The upper ends of the radius and ulna—the forearm bones—serve similarly, but it is in the humerus attachments and their muscle functions that most tennis elbow miseries develop.

At the lower end of the humerus, just above and to either side of its twin articulating knobs and its olecranon notch, are two bony projections, or protuberances, called epicondyles. If you cup one of your elbows, half-bent, in your opposite hand, you can readily feel these two protuberances with your fingers on both sides of your elbow. (The bony projection you feel at the back of your elbow is the spur of the ulna bone of your forearm, which is the olecranon process I have already described.) These protuberances get their name from the Latin *"condylus,"* which means knuckle, and, indeed, they feel like knuckles. When you go out to a restaurant and order pig's knuckles, it is these equivalents in the pig's leg bones that are delivered to your table.

The two epicondyles on either side of your elbow (they are, remember, protuberances on the sides of the lower end of the humerus and are not part of the joint itself) are called in medical terms the *lateral* epicondyle, meaning the projection, or knuckle, on the outside of the elbow, and the *medial* epicondyle, meaning the projection, or knuckle, on the inside. These two epicondyles serve as attaching points for the muscles that flex and extend your elbow and wrist. These muscles are the *flexor* and *extensor* muscles of your forearm.

THE ROLE OF THE MUSCLES AND TENDONS

When we get into muscles, things grow a bit more complicated. As I mentioned earlier, people tend to think of the muscles in their body as isolated and separately functioning components. I have shown how this image is inaccurate: there are hundreds of muscles in the body, all of which *interact* individually and in groups to perform the functions muscles are supposed to perform. The same is true with respect to particular regions of the body—the arm, for instance. In the arm there are dozens of muscles and muscle groups that interact to produce various movements. These muscles are not, as some imagine, separate, small entities each with its own isolated function or purpose. Rather, they resemble the cords of a thick hawser, overlapping for considerable distances throughout the arm and connecting to its bones at various points.

The arm is like the two leaves of a strap hinge, with the elbow as its joint. The upper arm is equivalent to the stationary leaf of the hinge, and the lower arm is the moveable leaf (the elbow does not provide the motion for the upper arm; this comes from the shoulder). When one wishes to move the lower arm, or forearm, in its straight hingelike motion, however, one calls upon the flexor and extensor muscles of the upper arm—the biceps and triceps, respectively—which are attached to the bones in the forearm portion of the elbow, as well as to the shoulder, to bring about the motion. The upper-arm muscles get help, of course, from the forearm muscles, but they do the main work.

Just as the upper-arm flexor and extensor muscles move the joint below them, the elbow, in a hingelike manner, so too do the flexor and extensor muscles of the forearm move the joint below *them* in an identical way. This joint is the wrist, and the flexors and extensors of the forearm are the principal muscles used in its flexion and extension, or downward and upward motions. The wrist, of course, is not a hinge joint in the sense that the elbow is; that is, it is capable of other directional motions besides straight hinge-movements, and I will get to these in a moment.

Insofar as the flexor and extensor muscles of the forearm control the up-and-down motions of the wrist, they serve the same functions as the flexors and extensors of the upper arm in moving the elbow. And just as the upper-arm muscles must be attached to the bones that are *on the other side* or *beyond* the joints they move, so too must *any* flexor or extensor be so attached.

In other words, the upper-arm flexors and extensors, to move the elbow, are attached to the bones below the elbow, the radius and the ulna. But they are also involved secondarily in the movement of the shoulder, so they are anchored to the bones on the other side of the shoulder joint as well.

Likewise, to move the wrist, the forearm flexors and extensors are attached to the bones below the wrist, and because they are also involved in the movement of the elbow, they must be anchored in the bone on the other side of the elbow joint. The bone they are attached to is the humerus, the bone of the upper arm. And the primary parts of the humerus they are attached to are the two epicondyles. The forearm extensor muscles are attached to the lateral, or outer, epicondyle; the forearm flexors to the medial, or inner, epicondyle.

The attachment, naturally, is made by tendons, as are all muscle-to-bone connections. And the tendons are named according to the muscles they attach. Thus, the tendon attaching the forearm extensor muscles to the outer, or lateral, epicondyle of your elbow is called the *extensor tendon;* the tendon attaching the forearm flexor muscles to the inner, or medial, epicondyle is called the *flexor tendon.*

It is the forearm *extensor muscles*, the *extensor tendon* and the *lateral epicondyle* with which we are concerned here, because these are the three components that conspire to produce the usual tennis elbow.

Before I focus entirely on these, however, let me answer a question that I'm sure occurred to you earlier when I said the elbow is only capable of one kind of motion—extension-flexion, or simple bending and unbending. You obviously have noticed when putting your arm through the several maneuvers it can make that you are able to rotate your forearm, and that by coupling this rotation with the various movements of your wrist, you can make your hand move in just about any direction you wish. Many of you are probably thereby convinced that your high degree of lower-arm mobility is due to a more-than-one-directional mobility in your elbow. Those of you who believe this no doubt wonder if I haven't been misleading you in describing the elbow's motion as being restricted to two straight directions, like that of a hinge.

Of course, I haven't been misleading you—the elbow joint *is* restricted to the straight, hingelike motion I have described. Your ability to rotate your forearm does not come from your elbow joint itself. It comes from other muscles in your forearm and from your wrist joint. If you lay your forearm flat on a table and rotate it from side to side, you'll notice that the motive force which enables you to do so comes from your wrist, not your elbow. You'll also notice the surface action of the muscles under the skin of your forearm as you rotate it. These are the muscles, called the forearm *pronator* and *supinator* muscles (because in medical terms the side-to-side rotation of the forearm is known as *pronation* and *supination*), that enable you to rotate your forearm.

Although the elbow joint itself doesn't move in these stationary rotations, the structures surrounding and supporting it, including the flexor and extensor muscles, and the appropriate tendons and ligaments, are involved in the pronation and supination of your forearm and wrist. Hence the forearm and wrist play a greater role in the development of the misery of tennis elbow than the elbow itself. Furthermore, as you have probably realized by now, tennis elbow is not actually an ailment of the interior of the elbow joint—something that many uninformed sufferers suspect—but of the outer and supporting structures of the joint, namely, the lateral epicondyle and the extensor tendon that attaches the forearm extensor muscles to that epicondyle.

Why, you ask, should the forearm and wrist be the culprits in tennis elbow? Especially when the pain you suffer is centered mainly in your elbow?

The answer is simple, really. Remember, the medical name for tennis elbow is lateral epicondylitis. This means an inflammation of the lateral epicondyle of the elbow. The inflammation comes about because the lateral epicondyle is the upper terminus, or point of attachment, of your forearm extensor muscles. Your forearm extensor muscles are what enable you to extend—raise or snap upward—your wrist. Every time you mis-strike a tennis ball with a racket, your stroke calls for a good deal of upward snap in your wrist. This upward snap, combined with the force of the ball hitting the racket, puts a higher than normal stress on your forearm extensor muscles. The stress radiates upward along these muscles and then suddenly comes to a stop at the point at which the extensor muscles are attached to your arm bone—at the lateral epicondyle. This sudden *stop of forces* produces a shock or trauma effect at the muscles' terminus. When the trauma is repeated a number of times, and when other factors are present, the repetition can cause an inflammation of the epicondyle in several ways, all of which will be painful.

What are these other factors? Well, here we get to the primary underlying causes of tennis elbow and the reason why the ailment can develop even in someone who doesn't play tennis.

As we have seen, your forearm consists of four main muscle groups—the extensors, the flexors, the pronators, the supinators. The extensors enable you to raise or snap your wrist and hand upward, and also to open your hand. Your flexors enable you to lower or snap your wrist and hand downward, and to close your hand. Your pronators enable you to rotate your forearm and wrist, turning the palm down. And your supinators enable you to rotate them so that the palm turns up.

Very seldom do we employ our hands in rigid, one-directional movements. Our hands and wrists are the most mobile parts of our body, and almost every action we take involves using them in a continually changing series of motions. Thus, the four primary muscle groups in our forearms are constantly interacting and working together to produce these varied motions.

We can assert up to this point, then, that tennis elbow is an inflammation of the site of attachment of the extensor muscles at the outside of the elbow, and that it directly involves the extensor muscles and their attaching tendon and indirectly involves the other muscles of the forearm. We can also say that tennis elbow comes about as a result of repeated traumatic overloads on the attachment site—the lateral epicondyle—due to any motion of the arm in which the forearm extensor muscles are required to do most of the work. For this reason, tennis elbow can develop in anyone; but because of several factors involved in the mechanics of the tennis stroke, it develops most frequently in tennis players.

THE PRECIPITATING CAUSES OF TENNIS ELBOW

There are three principal factors in tennis, and, to a lesser degree, in other racket sports, that create the conditions which lead to tennis elbow. The first is the *force of the speeding ball* as it meets the opposite-speeding racket. The second is the *dissipation of that force* through the arm. And the third is the ability of all the structures in the arm to *satisfactorily dissipate that force*.

The first two factors are invariables, that is, they always exist in tennis. The third is the all-important variable, and it depends on two further factors: (a) the point at which the ball is hit in relation to the arm; and (b) the ability of the muscles of the arm, especially the forearm muscles, to absorb excessive stresses that arise from faulty ball-arm relationship at the moment of impact. These two factors, unfortunately, are more often present than not in the recreational tennis player and are the primary villains in the development of tennis elbow.

What this means, in plainer English, is that the constant hitting of a tennis ball in an awkward or improper way, coupled with unconditioned forearm extensor muscles, will usually produce some form of tennis elbow. When these two factors are present, tennis elbow will almost invariably result. And it will frequently result when only one of the factors is present, particularly when the factor is weak or unconditioned extensor muscles.

Why the extensors? This should be obvious. Just about every stroke in tennis involves a sudden extension of the wrist. This is how the tennis player gets the snap into his or her shot. The forehand shot consists of a slight extension and supination of the wrist as the racket approaches the ball, then a sudden flexion and pronation as the arm follows through. The backhand shot consists of a flexion and pronation first, then an extension and supination as the racket meets the ball and the arm follows through. The serve demands wrist extension as the arm rotates to strike the ball, as does the overhead smash and just about every other stroke you can possibly make. Indeed, without wrist extension it is impossible for you to get either snap in your shot or spin on the ball. And every time you extend your wrist you must contract your forearm extensor muscles, thereby placing a "pull" or contraction force on the extensor tendon that attaches your extensor muscles to your elbow's lateral, or outside, epicondyle.

Such a contraction force under normal conditions —that is, conditions for which nature designed the extensor muscles and their tendon attachment—is easily absorbed by the extensor muscles and tendon. It is only when abnormal contractions occur on a relatively constant basis that trouble occurs. In the *ideal* tennis stroke, the wrist is in a "neutral" position when the racket meets the ball, that is, extension and supination have occurred, the wrist is straight, and flexion and pronation occur the moment after contact is made. But how many of us weekend athletes possess the ideal tennis stroke? Or, at least, how many of us are capable of executing it with any degree of consistency? Precious few, according to most of the professionals with whom I've discussed this matter.

Among the nearly 12 million Americans, 5 million Australians and almost 2 million Britons playing tennis today, there are perhaps 8,000 performers with exceptional talent—that is, with mechanically superior technique—and an elite group of about 400 men and women of world championship class. Although a very occasional case of tennis elbow will flare in someone from these two groups, the vast majority of complaints come from the 19 million-or-so recreational players in the three largest tennis-playing countries. This is not only because there are vastly more recreational players than full-time competitors but also because the unpolished player's anatomical distortions and improper techniques leave him more vulnerable to injury.

I had a conversation with the great Australian professional John Newcombe, just before he won the 1973 Forest Hills tennis championship. Newcombe told me that in his view the only permanent prescription for the prevention or elimination of tennis elbow is proper stroking technique. He said that in Australia he had cured numerous players of the ailment simply by teaching them the proper mechanics of the swing, which largely involves ensuring that the ball-racket-arm relationship is correct and that the wrist is in a neutral position at the moment of impact.

This is so apparent to common sense that it hardly seems worth noting. Yet, as in so many things in life, the common-sense items are often easiest to overlook. I have treated hundreds of tennis elbow patients who blame everything from poor rackets or "heavy" balls to air pollution or the alignment of their stars for their conditions. Like many of us in varying circumstances in our lives, they forget Cassius's famous admonition, "The fault, dear Brutus, is not in the stars. . . ."

There is no question that an improper stroke is the principal *precipitating cause* of tennis elbow. When most recreational tennis enthusiasts strike the ball, they do so with their wrists still in an extended position. Furthermore, as John Newcombe pointed out to me, the moment of impact comes at a time when their arms are either too far in front of their bodies or too far behind.

This combination of factors produces two events. The force of the ball hitting the racket sends an abnormal stress through the forearm extensor muscles, and this stress comes to an abrupt halt at the muscles' terminus in the extensor tendon and its insertion in the lateral epicondyle, causing a shock.

The second event exacerbates the first. When the arm is too far in front or too far behind the body at the moment of impact, it loses the support it would ordinarily get from the shoulder. Thus the stresses on the extensor muscles, which would ordinarily radiate further up the arm and be absorbed by the shoulder and the entire side of the body, have nowhere to go once they reach the lateral epicondyle of the elbow. The shock in this area is therefore compounded.

One reason why most professional and top-notch

amateur tennis players do not suffer from tennis elbow
is, although they occasionally must make an awkward
or off-balance shot, these shots are few and far between,
and the abnormal loads and stresses on their extensor
muscles are not constantly repeated. We weekenders,
however, are more likely to fall victim because we repeat the traumas to our lateral epicondyles through
repeated faulty stroke-impacts.

THE UNDERLYING CAUSES OF
TENNIS ELBOW

Another reason why most expert players do not
suffer from tennis elbow is because by playing as frequently as they do, they continually condition their
forearm muscles to absorb some of the overloads occa-
sioned by faulty stroking before these loads and stresses
reach the epicondyle area. And this brings us to the
underlying cause of tennis elbow—weak or unconditioned forearm musculature.

It is always very easy to identify professional or
full-time amateur tennis players, even when they are
not on the court. It is also easy to determine whether
they are right- or left-handed. All you have to do is look
at their forearms and compare one to the other.

Rod Laver, another great Australian champion, is
probably the most famous example of this. Laver is a
southpaw, and although he is a physically slight man,
his left forearm is huge, especially in relation to the
other parts of his body, particularly his right forearm.
Although I have never measured it personally, I have
read newspaper reports that claim his left forearm is
almost twice the diameter of his right.

This characteristic exists to some degree in all the top full-time players, women included, and goes a long way to account for the rarity of tennis elbow in these competitors. Their forearm muscles—their extensors, flexors, pronators and supinators—are all overdeveloped to a marked degree. These muscles are extraordinarily strong and supple and are superbly conditioned to withstand and absorb the traumatic overloads of awkward or off-balance shots.

Almost every case of tennis elbow I have seen in the past fifteen years has been suffered by an individual with insufficiently developed forearms. This is not to say that a person with strong and highly developed forearm muscles will be able to withstand the repeated traumas of a consistently poor swing without developing tennis elbow. But I can guarantee that the person with weak or poorly developed muscles is a prime candidate for the ailment.

Oversized forearms, however, are not invariably an indication of sufficient strength, nor are undersized forearms always an indication of weakness. There are hand-squeeze tests that measure the strength of forearm muscles—especially the extensors—and an individual with thin but supple forearms will often score higher than one with thick but flabby forearms. However, as a result of my observations over the years, I can say without fear of contradiction that weak or underdeveloped forearm muscles, whether flabby or thin, go hand-in-hand, so to speak, with tennis elbow. Indeed, they are the principal *underlying cause* of tennis elbow.

Why? The answer should be obvious by now. Weak or underdeveloped forearms muscles impose more of a shock-effect in what we doctors call the musculo-tendinous units of these muscles—the areas of their attachment to the bones. And since the forearm extensor muscles are the most frequently abused because of faulty wrist extension at the moment of impact in the tennis stroke, their musculo-tendinous unit, at the lateral epicondyle of the elbow, suffers the most frequent traumas. The repetition of this trauma in turn creates inflammation, either in the epicondyle alone, or in the epicondyle, extensor tendon, and muscle together. The inflammation is further brought about or aggravated by the mechanically bad relationship of the arm to the rest of the body during the moment of impact, creating even more intense stresses on the extensor muscles and more intense shocks to their musculo-tendinous unit.

There, then, are the fundamental causes of tennis elbow. But what exactly is tennis elbow? And how can it be cured and/or prevented from occurring?

THE EFFECTS OF TENNIS ELBOW

By now you should have a pretty good idea of what tennis elbow is. You should know that, constructed as it is, the elbow is predisposed to a concentration of forces at the lateral epicondyle, creating a fulcrum effect which, with excessive use of the forearm as a power source, produces an intrinsic overload in the extensor muscle group. You should also know that tennis is the one sport above all which, when played properly, uses the upper arm and shoulder as a power source and, when played improperly, uses the lower arm and wrist as a power source. In other words, properly played, tennis uses the entire body to generate the power behind its strokes; improperly played—that is,

the improper placement of the racket in relation to the
wrist and body at moment of impact—it puts almost the
entire burden of power on the forearm. The excess
stress that derives therefrom inevitably terminates in
the lateral epicondyle of the elbow.

The mechanics involved in this process can cause
a variety of tissue damages in the epicondyle region,
either singly or in combination. For instance, damage
may consist of only surface irritation to the epicondyle
itself where the extensor tendon ties into it. Or it may
encompass the epicondyle surface plus tears in the tissues of the tendon at or near its juncture with the epicondyle. Or it may further encompass tears in the tendon at or near its tie-in with the extensor muscles, and
might even involve tears in the muscle tissue itself.
Finally, and this is when tennis elbow can become a
permanent condition when not corrected, it might include a tearing away of a portion of the tendon from the
epicondyle's bony surface, or of a portion of the bone
itself. It can even involve the joint by pulling away part
of the capsule which encloses it.

In all these cases, mild to severe inflammation of
the affected parts is the result, and pain, mild to severe,
follows. The pain is centered in the outside point of the
elbow, the lateral epicondyle, and intensifies whenever
the elbow is moved, because in movement the extensor
muscles pull on the tendon, which in turn pulls on the
epicondyle. And when the extensor muscles are put to
normal use, such as in shaking hands, cutting meat,
brushing teeth, and so on, the discomfort becomes agonizing, sending sharp arrows of pain shooting down the
forearm's extensor muscles to the wrist. Of course,
when inflammation and pain progress to the agonizing
stage, tennis, and most other sports, are out of the question.

Tennis elbow is really a two-phase process, and because of this it tends to become chronic. The first phase is the repeated-trauma phase, which causes the initial inflammation. The trauma phase causes small swellings around the musculo-tendinous unit. Then, between episodes of tennis playing—when the victim is not subjecting his or her forearm and elbow to excess stresses—the extensor muscles tend to atrophy ever so slightly as the swelling spontaneously reduces. The atrophying process tends to further limit the already minimal elasticity of the extensor tendon. The next time out on the courts there is more stress and more trauma, and afterward more swelling and more atrophy. This process is repeated for several weeks or months until the victim has elbow pain all the time— on the courts and off. He or she now tends to avoid the natural elbow-forearm-wrist extension movements that cause pain in everyday life, thereby causing the extensor muscles to shrink, and placing a greater permanent pull on the extensor tendon as it attaches to the epicondyle. This pull, which derives from the shrunken muscles, is the second phase of tennis elbow and accounts for the continual elbow pain the victim experiences, even when he or she is not using the affected arm.

THE TREATMENT, CURE, AND PREVENTION OF TENNIS ELBOW

Now, the first treatment for tennis elbow is plain-and-simple rest. However, rest by itself is usually not enough, as the above example of the two phases illustrates. Rest will help reduce inflammation and pain in mild cases, but for the victim to return to tennis after the pain is gone, without doing anything to build up his or her extensor and associated forearm muscles, is to extend an open invitation to the tennis elbow to return immediately. This is because the atrophied extensor muscle will be that much more inclined to increase the tension on the extensor tendon and epicondyle. The result will be an even more painful tennis elbow than before.

This is a subject that perplexes a great many people who suffer athletic injuries or ailments. I have already hinted at it, but will state it in stronger terms here: no athletic injury or ailment will heal sufficiently to permit the enthusiast to resume his or her favorite athletic activities unless such healing is accompanied by a re-building and restrengthening of the structures sur-rounding the site of the injury or ailment. It is often a weakness in these structures that permits the ailment to develop in the first place; therefore, the structures must be not only rebuilt to their former strength, they should be rebuilt to a point well beyond their former strength to ensure against a recurrence of the ailment. *Prevention, truly, is the best medicine.*

Injuries and ailments are one of the hazards of athletic activity. The fact that they exist should not offset the benefits to be gained by participation in sports, but the risk of contracting them exists neverthe-less. The prudent athlete—weekend or fulltime—is aware of these risks and knows how to reduce them to a minimum. Most weekend athletes are not all that prudent. They wish to pack as much action as they can into the short time they have. They will often extend themselves beyond their bodies' capacity to withstand what would otherwise be endurable and nondamaging traumas. Moreover, they fail to condition the relevant parts of their bodies to endure these traumas, thereby making them more likely to receive damage.

Most professional athletes are much more prudent. They have to be, for it is through sports that they make their living. They appreciate the value of conditioning and know that without it their injuries and ailments would be much more frequent. And with the advent of sports medicine, they are beginning to appreciate the value not only of the healing process when they *are* injured, but of the rebuilding and double-strengthening of related structures as well. They are fast learning that this is the only way to prevent the recurrence of their injuries and ailments.

This axiom applies with no more validity to any other ailment than it does to tennis elbow. Rest, for the sake of healing, is only the beginning of treatment. Without a corresponding double-strengthening of the forearm extensor muscles, rest is practically worthless —at least for the individual who wants to continue playing tennis. And even then that's not enough. The tennis elbow victim should also take a sufficient number of lessons to teach him or her the proper way to stroke the ball—forehand, backhand, overhead, and all the shots between.

When these three stages—extended *rest*, then *muscle strengthening*, and *proper stroke-technique* learning—are completed, more likely than not a mild case of tennis elbow will disappear and not return. If that seems a great price to pay, remember that I said at the beginning of this book that no pleasure comes without a little sacrifice. Better a temporary pain in your pocketbook than a permanent pain in your elbow!

I can't tell you what's wrong with your tennis stroke or grip because I can't see them. You should submit them to the scrutiny of a qualified professional, and let him make the necessary alterations. I can tell you, however, that tennis-elbow causing defects occur in every stroke; and that if you have any of these defects you are more likely than not to develop a case of tennis elbow—if you haven't already.

Hitting backhands too far in front of your body with your wrist extended and your elbow bent, forces you to rely on your elbow and wrist snap to hit the ball. At the moment of contact, your forearm, from the elbow down to the wrist, becomes the focus of all the forces of both the speeding ball and the swinging racket; you, in effect, have no counterbalancing leverage, except for your forearm. And if the ball is not struck in the center of the racket, the force of the ball overcomes your forearm force, thereby compounding the overload in your extensor muscles and doubling, or even trebling, what is already an abnormal overload because of your faulty position in relation to the ball. Once the overload reaches the bent fulcrum of your elbow it has nowhere further to go because your body —your upper arm, shoulder, back, etc.—are too far forward to absorb the force.

Similar dynamics hold true for a backhand that is stroked too far behind you, with similar bodily configuration. In this case you reduce the movement of your shoulder and upper arm in order to "catch" the ball before it gets past you. The swing is all forearm and wrist, with exaggerated pronation and flexion at the start, then equally exaggerated extension and supination to get some snap into the shot. Usually the moment of impact comes as you abruptly snap or extend your wrist, and the result is a tremendous unabsorbed overload on your unprotected extensor muscles. And trying to put a special spin on the ball further complicates things.

In any tennis shot the forearm should be the source

of control, *not the source of power.* The power should come from the motion and rotation of the shoulder coupled with body-weight transfer. Thus, an ideal backhand is executed with the front shoulder down and rotating as you shift your weight from back to front foot. You should plan to strike the ball just as it reaches your front foot, not out ahead of it, not behind it. You should be at approximately a right angle to the ball with your trunk leaning toward the net, and your elbow and wrist firm and fairly straight.

The same general principles apply to the other strokes in tennis—it's mostly a matter of body position. But my purpose in this book is not to give you tennis lessons. Reading how to properly execute various strokes can never be the same as having them demonstrated and then practicing them until perfect, or near perfect. And anyway, I am not as qualified to instruct you as a professional in the field. So I'll leave the instruction to the professionals, with the strong recommendation that you consult one—for learning correct stroking technique is one of the most important factors in eliminating tennis elbow. But only consult one *after* you've given your elbow sufficient rest to effect healing of the lateral epicondyle and its related musculo-tendinous area, and *after* you have faithfully worked on the task of restoring and strengthening your forearm extensor muscles.

EXERCISES FOR TENNIS ELBOW

In this regard there is a very simple exercise you should do daily to rebuild, strengthen or condition your forearm extensor muscles. You can either go out and buy a small, adjustable-weight dumbbell to assist you or use progressively heavier books from your bookshelves. I would recommend the dumbbell purchase, since this device is easier to handle than books.

Exercise 1.   Forearm Extensor Curl

Sit in a chair and elevate the thigh on the same side of your body as the arm you'll be exercising. (Elevate your thigh by resting your foot on a block or footstool, four to six inches high). Take the dumbbell or book (about two pounds in weight to begin with) in your hand. Place your forearm (elbow to wrist) along the length of your thigh, with your hand, palm down, extending past your kneecap. With the palm of your hand still down, lift (extend) your wrist as high as it will go without raising your forearm. Hold your wrist extension at maximum, pressing your forearm against your thigh, for a slow count of five, then release. Work up to thirty repetitions, and when you can do thirty comfortably with two pounds, increase the weight to three pounds and work up to thirty repetitions again. When you can comfortably achieve thirty repetitions at three pounds, increase the weight again to four pounds, and so on up.

This is an exercise you should do twice a day, every day, if you have, or have had, tennis elbow and want to continue playing tennis without pain. You should not begin it, however, until you have rested your elbow for a while or had it treated by a physician, so that the exercise itself does not produce elbow pain. It is also an exercise you should do at least every other day if you are a weekend tennis player, are convinced your stroking techniques are not on a par with a professional's, and have not yet suffered from tennis elbow.

This exercise is prophylactic, that is, it helps prevent an ailment from occurring. It can also be therapeutic, which is to say it can actually contribute to the healing process by taking the inherent strain off the musculo-tendinous area of the elbow and reducing the inflammation. There are three other exercises you can do almost anytime and anywhere, without the need for weights, that are also beneficial.

Exercise 2.   Isometric Forearm Extension
Hold your arm fully extended in front of your body. Fully extend (pull back) your fingers and wrist. Hold for a slow count of five, then release. Repeat fifty times.

Exercise 3.   Double Isometric Forearm Extension
Hold your arm as in Exercise 2 and make a fist. Place your opposite hand over the fist and cup it firmly. Then, while extending (raising) your wrist-fist, push down with the cupped hand, exerting as strong a counter-force as possible. Hold for a slow count of five, then release. Twenty repetitions.

Exercise 4.   Tennis Ball Squeeze
Hold your arm fully extended in front of your body with your hand, palm down, gripping a tennis ball. Squeeze the ball as hard as you can, hold for a slow count of five, then relax your hand. Fifty repetitions.

These exercises, one or another, should be done a few times every day. Coupled with learning the proper ways to stroke, they will go a long way towards preventing the occurrence—or recurrence—of tennis elbow.

FURTHER TREATMENTS

If your tennis elbow, or epicondyle inflammation, is of the mild variety, the treatment I have just outlined should work well. However—and unfortunately— many cases of this ailment are not mild. They are severe; they cause intense pain in the arm, make many normal everyday activities agonizing to perform, and make tennis and many other sports impossible to play. When tennis elbow reaches this stage, it requires medical treatment.

Before I get to medical treatment, let me say that it has been fairly well determined by researchers that tennis elbow is principally an ailment of adulthood, and it may even be connected to the aging process. The problem rarely affects people under twenty, and the large majority of its victims are over thirty. The reason for this is probably twofold. First, youngsters are usually much more active in their daily lives than adults, and their overall muscle tone is kept at a higher peak. Second, as we age, our connective tissues become less elastic, and have less "rebound;" we therefore lose a certain amount of resilience, which predisposes the susceptible areas to damage. We all know that the older we get, the slower our recuperative powers become.

No one knows exactly what biochemical changes occur in our elbows and forearms to increase the incidence of tennis elbow in proportion to age, but I suspect that much of it has to do with the fact that our elbows, as other parts of our bodies, suffer a lessening of their recuperative powers. When we are young our elbows are able to spontaneously recuperate from the repeated shocks of faulty tennis stroking, but as we age they lose that ability and the shock factor eventually prevails. Also, many tennis enthusiasts have not taken up the sport until their late twenties or early thirties. Thus they have started with forearms and elbows that have not been conditioned to repeated traumas.

The medical treatment of severe tennis-elbow conditions follows a progression. Doctors generally try to be as conservative as possible in their treatment at first. If an ailment does not respond to the most conservative form of treatment, they will then propose progressively more radical procedures until the problem is overcome. The most radical, of course, is surgery, which has a high degree of success, and which I'll discuss in a moment.

The twin goals of medical treatment are to relieve the inflammation and pain of tennis elbow and to prevent its recurrence. Unfortunately, the conservative approach, although it can achieve the first goal rather readily, has a very low success rate in achieving the second. This is because it must rely so heavily on the patient's motivation and self-discipline to strengthen his or her forearm muscles and to learn to hit a tennis ball correctly.

It is no secret among doctors that once patients are relieved of pain, they tend to forget about the conditions that brought it about and make little or no effort to prevent its recurrence. A physician can only provide so much treatment and therapy. He can diagnose a condition and prescribe the measures required to reverse it as rapidly as possible, so that the patient is relieved of pain, discomfort, and anxiety. He can also

recommend measures the patient should take to prevent recurrence—whether they be to quit smoking, to
stop eating candy, to sleep on a hard bed, or, as in the
case of tennis elbow, to exercise the forearm regularly
and learn the proper strokes. What he can't do is force
the patient to follow his advice, and this is why so many
tennis-elbow victims become regular visitors to their
doctors' offices.

The primary objective of treatment is, as I have
said, to reduce the inflammation, for it is the inflammation in the epicondyle region that causes the pain of
tennis elbow. The most conservative way of reducing
inflammation is to apply ice directly to the lateral epicondyle. Aspirin, because it seems to have an anti-
inflammatory effect, will also be prescribed for patients
who do not have aspirin-sensitive stomachs. And, of
course, a period of rest sufficient to allow for healing of
the damaged elbow parts.

The secondary objective of treatment is to bring
about an improvement in the tissues of the distressed
elbow. This is where the forearm exercise program
comes in. No matter what kind of primary treatment
the victim receives—from the most conservative to the
most radical—the improvement of the affected connective tissues of the elbow through exercise will *always* be
required. So, if you have tennis elbow, you must make
up your mind to commit yourself wholeheartedly to the
proposition that you, and only you, can overcome it in
the end. If you continue to play tennis with anything
less than such a commitment, you will then find yourself a victim of continuing, chronic, and increasingly
more severe tennis elbow. I'm afraid I cannot stress this
enough.

A third objective of treatment consists in bringing

about a diminution of the moments of force at the forearm when playing tennis. This means, of course, improving your stroke. You must learn to utilize fully the power inherent in a proper transfer of body weight, and in the shoulder muscles. You should use the forearm for *racket control only*, not for power itself. In addition, you would be well advised to make sure you are using the proper racket. A light, flexible racket—conventionally strung (fifty-pound tension) with sixteen-gauge gut—is, in my experience, the easiest on the forearm. Appropriate grip size is very important as well —the smaller the grip, the better.

Returning to the primary objective of treatment, if simple ice-rest-aspirin therapy doesn't work, the next step up the ladder is cortisone.

CORTISONE

Now I'm sure most of you have heard about cortisone-injection treatment for tennis elbow, and the likelihood is that many of you with this ailment have had it and have been disappointed to discover that it didn't work. Your disappointment is undoubtedly due to the fact that you were led to believe that cortisone can "cure" tennis elbow. This, of course, is a myth. Cortisone treatments don't cure, they are merely an effective and rapid way to reduce or eliminate inflammation.

By using cortisone, a physician can reduce elbow pain and inflammation almost overnight, thereby providing a patient with immediate relief and the opportunity to begin improving the affected elbow and forearm tissues through exercise that much sooner. Why, then, you might ask, isn't cortisone used right away all the time?

The answer is that cortisone doesn't automatically work for everyone, and it can also have unpleasant side effects for certain people. It is a steroid drug and must be administered with great care. While it will usually reduce inflammation at the epicondyle, too much of it, repeated too often, can cause a certain amount of degeneration in the bone tissues of the elbow, leaving the patient worse than before.

When administered properly, though, cortisone can be of great help in achieving the permanent relief of tennis elbow, especially when healing is permitted to take place, and the strengthening of muscle and other involved tissues is faithfully pursued by the patient. It is administered by injection directly into the lateral epicondyle and extensor tendon of the elbow along with a local anesthetic.

After the anesthetic wears off, the patient might experience a pain in his elbow that is even more intense than his ordinary tennis-elbow pain, but this will last only for a few hours. Thereafter, the pain will rapidly diminish to nothing; not only will the pain of the injection disappear, but so too will most, if not all, of the pain of tennis elbow.

Another approach to chemical therapy is the use of a drug called butazolidin. This can be used separately or in conjunction with cortisone; it has a similar anti-inflammatory effect but takes longer to work because it is ingested orally over a period of a few days to a week. The anti-inflammatory agents in this compound get into the blood-supply system, and when they reach the inflamed area they go to work.

Because the drug is carried by the blood, it too can have dangerous side effects, especially in elderly people or in individuals with gastrointestinal, liver, and other organic problems. It therefore must be selectively administered, and the patient should be carefully monitored for deleterious side effects both while on the drug and afterwards.

Let me say again that although cortisone and butazolidin can be very effective aids in the medical treatment of tennis elbow, they are not, in themselves, cures. The only cure for tennis elbow is rest, followed by rehabilitation of the affected muscle, tendon, and bone tissues. Because many victims of tennis elbow lack sufficient motivation and self-discipline to achieve such rehabilitation, tennis elbow will often recur and become chronic weeks or months after cortisone and/or butazolidin therapy has seemed to work.

In these cases another round of such drugs is administered and the same process usually repeats itself. It can be safely said that if tennis elbow continues to recur after more than two injections of cortisone, it has become chronic. Cortisone, or butazolidin, will continue to provide temporary relief, but the patient will find his ailment returning sooner and sooner each time. He will now be on an expensive "treatment treadmill" when he could be saving himself a lot of money by either giving up tennis or by really resolving to go to work on strengthening his arm. Since he or she understandably cannot bear giving up tennis, and should not, arm strengthening exercises are the only alternative— short of surgery, of course, but even surgical correction of the condition requires arm strengthening.

ELBOW SURGERY

With the rapidly increasing incidence of tennis elbow, there has been a corresponding increase in tennis-elbow surgery over the past few years. In one sense, surgery, being the most radical form of treatment, is the least desirable because it is the most expensive, requires hospitalization, and entails a long period of recuperation before tennis activities can be resumed. Yet because of the success such surgery has had, in another sense it is the most desirable treatment in cases of severe or frustratingly chronic tennis elbow.

There are several procedures used in tennis-elbow surgery. The most common consists of making a small incision along the line of the extensor tendon where it connects the extensor muscle group to the lateral epicondyle. The surgeon, using tried-and-proven techniques, then releases the tension on the tendon by cutting it and letting it slide away from the epicondyle. This allows new tendinous tissue to grow and reattach to the epicondyle, but in a much less taut fashion. He then trims down the epicondyle itself by scraping away excess granulation created by the inflammation.

Postsurgical treatment includes immobilizing the elbow and lower arm for a short period of time followed by physical therapy to restore the extensor and associated forearm muscles to their original strength. Once the patient is able to use his elbow freely again, he should then proceed to full-scale exercises, such as the ones I have detailed, to develop even greater strength and flexibility in the forearm. Eventually, tennis can be resumed.

Surgery will in most cases "cure" a severe tennis elbow, but it does not prevent it from returning. The extensor muscles are still, for the most part, attached to the epicondyle, and although the fulcrum effect has been reduced, a return to bad stroking habits, plus a failure to strengthen the forearm muscles, can lead to a complete repetition of the process that brought the original ailment about.

ELBOW BRACES

Many doctors recommend, either with or without surgery, that tennis enthusiasts with elbow problems use *counterforce braces* or *forearm compression bands* when playing. A counterforce brace is a bulky affair that slips onto your arm above and below your elbow and has articulating struts in between. It allows you a certain amount of elbow mobility but prevents full elbow extension when swinging at a ball, thereby reducing the overload of even improperly executed shots.

Forearm compression bands are two-to-three-inch-wide straps that tighten snugly over your forearm just below the elbow. The theory of these is that by compressing your extensor muscles near the greatest source of trouble, they reduce the tension on the tendon fibers that originate from the lateral epicondyle.

Both of these devices can be effective for relieving the existing pains in tennis elbow while playing, especially when used in conjunction with aspirin or some other mild analgesic, but they are useless in preventing a worsening of the ailment. Indeed, I strongly advise against their use because they tend to create more problems than they solve. By taking up part of the work designed for the extensor muscles themselves, these devices contribute to a further weakening, rather than strengthening, of the elbow and its associated muscles. Their continued use can therefore actually contribute to the conditions that produce tennis elbow. I would only recommend a counterforce brace for elderly people who cannot tolerate cortisone, or for people whom surgery has not helped but who still have an overwhelming desire to continue playing tennis. In these cases I feel that the exercise-benefits of tennis far outweigh the alternative of having to give the game up, and that counterforce braces are a happy, if not ideal, compromise.

SPONTANEOUS REMISSION

If it's any consolation to some of you, tennis elbow will sometimes disappear on its own, without any treatment, as suddenly as it began. This is known in medicine as "spontaneous remission," and I wish I could tell you why it happens. But I can't.

Nobody knows why spontaneous remission occurs; we can only guess that through some unidentified mechanism of nature, the elbow rehabilitates itself. Most cases of spontaneous remission occur in individuals who keep playing tennis despite their pain: it is possible that by continuing to play, the individual's forearm muscles gradually strengthen to a point where they are able to withstand the repeated overloads and traumas of faulty shot making. Many tennis pros subscribe to this theory, and one well-known teaching pro in New York strongly advises his pupils to "play through" their episodes of tennis elbow. I doubt that this is the best medical advice to be given. But I know many game people who are willing to follow it, so rabid is their enthusiasm for tennis. Of course, the best way to achieve spontaneous remission is to learn the proper stroking techniques, and perhaps this is what the "play-through-it" teaching pro has in mind.

Professional or amateur, most tennis addicts with tennis elbow are determined to keep playing at any cost. Some go so far as to relearn the game with their other arm, only to develop a case of "double" tennis elbow. Others bravely endure the pain that each swing of the racket brings. One buff in my neighborhood has even found a bright side to his affliction. "When I hit a backhand," he explains, "I often let loose with a scream of pain. My opponent is usually so disconcerted that he can't return the shot."

Better than turning your ailment to the purposes of court psychology, however, is getting rid of it—or at least reducing it to the point where it no longer materially interferes with your enjoyment of the game. I have hinted at, suggested, implored, and stated outright on a dozen occasions throughout this chapter where the greatest chances of success lie and how to best achieve that success. The rest, as I have also said with equal frequency, is up to you. In the end, it can only be the victim who can conquer his or her tennis elbow.

THROWER'S ELBOW

Many of you might guess that thrower's elbow is somehow the opposite of tennis elbow. Not true. In the first place, thrower's elbow can also be a form of tennis elbow. Although the pain and inflammation occur on the inside of the elbow in this ailment, the mechanics and causes of the condition are similar to those of conventional tennis elbow.

If you'll go back to my discussion of the anatomy of

the elbow, you'll recall that I described the upper-arm
bone, the humerus, as having an outer *and* an inner
epicondyle at its lower terminus (see Fig. 9). Lateral
epicondylitis, or tennis elbow, is an inflammation of the
outer epicondyle caused by the excessive pull and
stretch of the forearm extensor muscles where they
attach to the lateral epicondyle through the intermedi-
ary of the extensor tendon, correct?

Well, medial epicondylitis—commonly called
thrower's elbow because it occurs mostly in baseball
pitchers and football passers—is an inflammation of the
inner epicondyle of the elbow, the *underlying causes*
of which are similar to the underlying causes of lateral
epicondylitis, even though the *precipitating causes* are
different. The only significant difference between the
two lies in the fact that because the ulnar nerve, one of
the major nerves of the arm, passes much closer to the
inner epicondyle than to the outer, medial epicondylitis can be infinitely more painful and debilitating than
lateral epicondylitis.

Just as the extensor muscles of the forearm attach
to the lateral epicondyle, so do the forearm's flexor
muscles attach to the medial epicondyle. Recall if you
will my description of the interrelationship and interac-
tion of all four principal muscle groups in the forearm:
the extensors, the flexors, the supinators, the pronators.

The extensors and supinators work most closely in
conjunction when the wrist and/or fingers are extended (raised) and the forearm and wrist are rotated
in a palm up direction. The flexors and pronators work
most closely together when the wrist and/or fingers are
flexed (lowered) and the forearm and wrist are rotated
palm downward. But there are many other combinations of movement possible, too, such as extending the

wrist while pronating the forearm, or flexing the wrist
while extending the fingers and supinating the forearm. So—all four muscle groups are in constant inter-
play.

The flexor muscles and their attachment to the
medial epicondyle are the chief villains in medial epicondylitis, and it is for this reason that the ailment can
occur in tennis players as well as in those who use their
arms to throw. The affliction comes about through repeated excessive strains and overloads on the flexor
muscles, and through the continual, unrelieved traumas they create at the site of their terminal attachment
to the elbow, the medial epicondyle.

In weekend tennis players, medial epicondylitis is
not nearly as common as lateral epicondylitis, but it is
considerably more devastating when it does occur. It is
not so common because there are only one or two faulty
strokes in tennis that place greater stress on the flexor
muscles of the forearm than on the extensors. These
strokes are forehand shots that are hit early, or in front
of the mid-line of the body, bringing about sudden wrist
snap (flexion and pronation) to compensate, and service
or overhead smash shots which, due to faulty timing,
cause the wrist to be hyperflexed at the moment of
impact. Of course, attempts to put excessive topspin on
the ball also cause hyperflexion and hyperpronation
whose stresses, when unabsorbed by the shoulder, terminate as shocks in the medial epicondyle.

It is this flexion-pronation-to-achieve-spin factor
which leads to the most frequent occurrence of medial
epicondylitis and tells the story of why it is more commonly associated with those who throw. Not many of us
indulge in track-and-field events as a form of recreational or weekend athletic activity, so that pretty well

leaves out of our discussion such throwing motions as are involved in shotputting, the discus, and the javelin.

Many of us do play touch football, softball, and baseball, however, and in all three of these sports the object when throwing the ball is to put spin on it. The football passer seeks to produce speed, trajectory, and distance by means of the spiral. The baseball pitcher seeks to produce speed and a sudden change of direction by imparting spin to the ball as it leaves his hand. So does the softball pitcher. And the fielders in both these sports are often required to throw hard and fast while off balance. All of these maneuvers bring the flexor and pronator muscles of the forearm intensely into play. And when these muscles aren't up to the repeated stresses placed on them, thrower's elbow, or medial epicondylitis, will often be the result.

For graphic evidence of how intensely involved the forearm flexors and extensors are in the act of throwing, the next time you see a slow-motion instant replay of a quarterback, pitcher, or outfielder in the act of delivering the ball, carefully note the position of his hand and wrist once the ball has left his fingers. You will see that his hand and wrist are in the extreme "down" and "turned-in" positions—that is, they are hyperflexed and hyperpronated.

The stresses become compounded in pitchers who throw curveballs and screwballs. A curveball requires sudden extension and supination of the wrist to impart spin, following by equally abrupt flexion and pronation in the follow-through. The screwball's spin is the reverse of the curve's; thus, the stresses on the arm of the screwball pitcher are hyperflexion and hyperpronation all the way through the motion of the arm as it releases the ball.

This is why it is so important for pitchers, throwers, and passers to warm their arms up gradually before engaging in any serious throwing. If they don't, the strains on their forearm flexor and pronator muscles, through the natural act of throwing, will soon tell in their elbows.

But they are professional athletes, and are expected to know these things. Weekend athletes, on the other hand, often don't. I can't count the times I've seen touch-football passers start right off in a game, without having warmed up, trying to throw sixty-yard "bombs." And how many times have you seen baseball or softball enthusiasts come right into a contest and start throwing clothesline strikes from the outfield or spinning nifty curves from the mound without having properly warmed up and stretched their arm muscles? I know the number of thrower's elbow victims must be countless because I get many of them in my office.

NERVE IMPINGEMENT

Chronic inflammation in the medial epicondyle region has an added danger that lateral epicondylitis generally doesn't and which makes its avoidance even more desirable. This is the fact that it can lead to ulnar-nerve impingement or entrapment.

There are three principal nerves that travel down your arm, pass across your elbow, and, by means of complex series of branches, sensitize the muscles and other tissues of your forearm, wrist, and hand. These are: the *radial* nerve (so called because it adjoins the radius bone), the *median* nerve (because it travels through the center of the forearm between the radius and the ulna), and the *ulnar* nerve (because it adjoins the ulna bone).

You will recall that the ulna is the bone that forms the inside part of your forearm. The ulnar nerve descends through the upper arm, passes through the elbow a hair's breadth beneath the medial epicondyle of the humerus, and then continues on down along the ulna. In passing just inside the medial epicondyle, the ulnar nerve becomes subject to any slight variations in the epicondyle's shape.

A simple illustration of how easily the ulnar nerve is affected by the medial epicondyle is an experience we have all gone through on more than one occasion: hitting what we call our "funny bone." When we accidentally strike the inside of our elbow against something hard, we experience the strange sensation, which lasts for only a few moments, of losing control of our little and ring fingers and experiencing a painful tingling along the course of the nerve.

What we have done, of course, is struck and momentarily shocked our medial epicondyle. We call this our "funny bone" for the obvious reason that the epicondyle is a protuberance of the humerus. What occurs is that the blow to the epicondyle suddenly compresses or "pinches" our ulnar nerve, causing both the pain we feel at the site and the numbness and loss of control we temporarily experience in our arm's lower extremities.

The same thing can occur during medial epicondylitis. Although it comes about in a more gradual way, inflammation of the epicondyle can cause scarring and, therefore, slight alterations in its shape, which in turn press on or pinch the ulnar nerve. As the compression of the nerve continues it can eventually cause entrapment. The sensitizing impulses carried by the nerve into the lower arm will become partially or completely blocked, causing chronic numbness and loss of control over those muscles of the forearm, wrist and hand that are dependent upon the ulnar nerve. You can see, then, that medial epicondylitis, or thrower's elbow, despite its association with the "funny bone," is no laughing matter.

TREATMENT OF THROWER'S ELBOW

The treatment, prevention, and cure of thrower's elbow are very similar to those prescribed for tennis elbow. Because of the possibility of ulnar nerve entrapment, however, and also because medial epicondylitis is more likely to lead to eventual arthritis* of the elbow than is lateral epicondylitis, it is often wiser to proceed immediately to surgery in cases of severe thrower's elbow. Again, surgery consists of releasing tension on the flexor tendon and removing any loose bony material around the epicondyle, which might threaten the ulnar nerve.

Prevention, of course, is what we really like to see, and most doctors will insist that victims, or potential victims, of thrower's elbow pursue a series of exercises designed to strengthen the flexor muscles. When conditioned, these muscles are in a better position to absorb some of the shocks of hyperflexion rather than letting

---

*I will not deal directly with arthritis in this book, but I will mention it off and on. Arthritis is an inflammation in any joint of the body and is brought about by simple wear and tear on the contacting joint surfaces, and by the presence of bone chips and spurs that interfere with normal joint function. Its primary causes are unknown at this time, as is its cure.

them all be absorbed by the medial epicondyle. These exercises are similar to the exercises I outlined earlier for tennis elbow. Because they are designed to strengthen the flexors rather than the extensors, however, they include a few differences in technique.

Exercise 1.   Forearm Flexor Curl

Sit on a chair and elevate the thigh on the same side of your body as the arm you'll be exercising. (Elevate your thigh by resting your foot on a block or footstool four to six inches high.) Take a dumbbell, book, or some other easily graspable object (about two pounds in weight to begin with) in your hand. Place your forearm (elbow to wrist) along the length of your thigh, with your hand—*palm up*—extending past your kneecap. With the palm of your hand still up, lift (flex) your wrist as high as it will go without raising your forearm. Hold your wrist flexion at maximum, pressing your forearm against your thigh, for a slow count of five—then relax and return your wrist to the neutral position. Work up to thirty repetitions, and when you can do thirty comfortably with two pounds, increase the weight to three pounds and work up to thirty repetitions again. When you can comfortably achieve thirty repetitions with three pounds, increase the weight again to four pounds, and so on up.

You should perform this exercise twice a day if you suspect that you have thrower's elbow, or even if you don't have any symptoms but engage in throwing sports periodically. In addition to being preventive, this exercise, like its extensor equivalent, is also therapeutic —it can actually contribute to healing by taking the inherent strain off the musculo-tendinous area of the inside part of your elbow and thereby reducing the inflammation of your medial epicondyle.

As with the forearm extensor exercises, there are several other useful flexor exercises you can do as you move about engaging in your ordinary, everyday activities. These are isometric exercises, and because they require no weights, you can perform them anywhere, anytime. Trying to flex your wrist against a stationary object such as a wall or door is one. Flexing your wrist while squeezing a ball is another. Flexing your wrist while rotating your forearm is still another. At first you will find that your forearm tires easily. But as your muscles gain strength, the fatigue factor will diminish. This is a good sign that the exercises are having a beneficial effect.

A final word about the elbow—I cannot emphasize strongly enough the importance of properly warming up your forearm muscles before engaging in tennis or throwing sports. To walk onto a court and start hitting balls at full speed, or to trot onto a football field and start throwing long, hard passes without first gradually warming up your arm muscles, is tantamount to elbow suicide. If your muscles are *not* gradually warmed up and stretched they will be in no position to absorb the abnormal stresses, forces, and loads imposed on them by strenuous, and sometimes violent, unsupported arm movements. And if your forearm muscles are weak or underdeveloped, you're putting yourself—and especially your elbow—in double jeopardy. So do yourself the biggest of all favors—before starting tennis or a game in which you'll be throwing a ball: warm up!

5

YOUR KNEE MISERIES
–TRICK OR TREAT!

You are sitting in an elegant restaurant coolly ordering a bottle of wine under the admiring gaze of your comely dinner companion and the critical eye of the sommelier. As you debate with yourself the virtues of a Chateau Margaux '61 as against those of the Haut-Brion '59, you shift on your chair and cross one leg over the other—a posture you reflexively settle into whenever you are about to make a big decision. As you do so, all thoughts of fine wines and comely dinner companions are suddenly wrenched from your mind. You turn pale and let out a mighty screech; then you proceed to upset the perfectly laid dining table in your haste to leap to your feet. The entire restaurant falls into a hush, and all eyes turn to watch as you awkwardly hop about on one leg, grasping your knee, and moaning in pain.

Or you are dashing for a taxi on a busy street corner, your arms laden with gifts and parcels from the afternoon's Christmas-shopping expedition. You are just a step or two away from the cab when you suddenly sprawl ingloriously onto the pavement. Your packages go every which way, and your skirt flies immodestly over your head, but you can think of nothing but the pain in your knee as you writhe on the ground trying to keep from passing out.

Or you are a stage star, and the scene calls for you to glide silently across a darkened room and burgle the contents of a sleeping woman's jewel chest. When you make your entrance the theater turns deathly still, and the audience waits in rapt anticipation. As you slowly make your way across the stage, each step you take produces a clicking sound that reverberates through the hushed theater. The entire illusion of stealth and impending drama is fractured, and the audience bursts into laughter. You stop, perplexed, and stare down at your knee—the villain in this unexpected turn of events.

Such incidents as these happen thousands of times a day all across the country. Knees "go out," or "lock," or do other strange things with little regard for time or place. If you have what is commonly called a "trick knee" (for that is what is generally behind most complaints about the knee), such incidents can occur anywhere, anytime—while you're in bed or on a dance floor, driving a car or playing a sport.

With respect to weekend athletic miseries, the knee is the second most frequently affected part of the body after the elbow. The knee is to the legs as the elbow is to the arms—it is the most crucial joint in our lower extremities, the joint which lets us perform the many movements our legs are capable of, which enables us to play the many sports we do.

Just as its function in the leg is similar to the elbow's function in the arm, anatomically the knee resembles the elbow in many ways. This is because at one time in our evolutionary history we walked on all fours, and our knees and elbows were more-or-less the same joint.

Like the elbow, the knee is an articulating hinge joint that allows motion in only one plane—flexion and extension, or bending and straightening. Also like the elbow, it is a joint composed of the conjunction of one large upper bone and two smaller lower bones, and comes equipped with the same kind of condyles, tendons, ligaments, muscles, and other tissue components that hold the elbow together. However, it is a considerably more complex joint than the elbow. And because it has so many more parts and is subject to more intensive stresses—due to the weight-bearing factor—a lot more can go wrong with it.

The ailment of the knee that occurs with the greatest frequency—it is the equivalent of lateral epicondylitis of the elbow because of the widespread misery it produces—is torn cartilage (the proper name for which, as I noted earlier, is *meniscus*). But torn cartilage is only the beginning. Torn cartilage often occurs in association with tears in one or more of the ligaments of the knee, which produce instability in the joint and account for a great many of the trick knees that hamper us.

"Trick knee" can mean different things to different people. It can mean the knee suddenly giving away when full weight is placed on it while walking, running, descending stairs, and the like. It can mean the knee "locking" in a certain position. Or it can mean a variety of strange sensations in the knee during normal joint articulation. Although the symptoms can vary, trick knee, whatever its particular manifestation, is generally caused by a torn cartilage, torn ligaments, or a combination of both.

I will explain the mechanics of trick knee in a moment, but before I do I should note that there are several other sports-associated ailments of the knee that can also cause chronic pain and misery. Among them are *patellar bursitis,* lately known as "surfer's knee," *patellar tendinitis,* known in the sports world as "jumper's knee," *patellar chondromalacia,* sometimes called "dancer's knee," and that age-old affliction known as "water on the knee," which has nothing to do with swimming and is not really water on the knee at all, but fluid within the knee joint resulting from inflammations of the joint's internal lubricating mechanisms. I shall explain these afflictions further along in this chapter.

TRICK KNEE

As in the case of tennis elbow, in order to best understand the causes and mechanics of trick knee it is desirable to understand something about the architecture of the joint in which it occurs. By now you have already gotten a sense of hinge-joint construction through my discussion of the elbow and its anatomy, so understanding your knee's architecture should be a bit more easy—despite the fact that although the two joints have many similarities, the knee is a bit more complex, with several more parts to worry about.

THE BONES OF THE KNEE

Skeletally, the knee is formed by the vertical joining of the thigh bone, the *femur*, to the two bones of the lower leg, the *tibia* and the *fibula*. In the design of the leg the femur can be considered the equivalent of the humerus, the long upper bone of the arm. Similarly, the tibia is the equivalent of the radius, the larger bone of the forearm, and the fibula is comparable to the ulna, the smaller forearm bone.

You will recall that in the construction of the elbow the humerus joins directly with the radius *and* the ulna by means of projections that fit into one another. Well, here we come to the first major dissimilarity between the knee and the elbow. In the knee, the thigh bone, or femur, *does not* connect directly with both lower-leg bones; it connects only with the larger one, the tibia.

At its lower end, the thigh bone is very similar to the upper-arm bone in its configuration; that is, it broadens out and forms into knuckles, two outer knobs and a center notch.

At its upper end, the larger of the two lower-leg bones, the tibia, widens and flattens into a corresponding configuration. At the very end of the tibia there are two condyles—inner and outer—with a projecting ridge separating them. This ridge fits into the center notch of the lower end of the thigh bone, and the flat surfaces of the two condyles fit against the rounded surfaces of the two projecting knobs—also called condyles—of the thigh bone's lower end. This conjunction of surfaces constitutes the skeletal design of the knee joint.

The fibula, the smaller bone of the lower leg, plays no part in the knee joint itself, as does the ulna in the

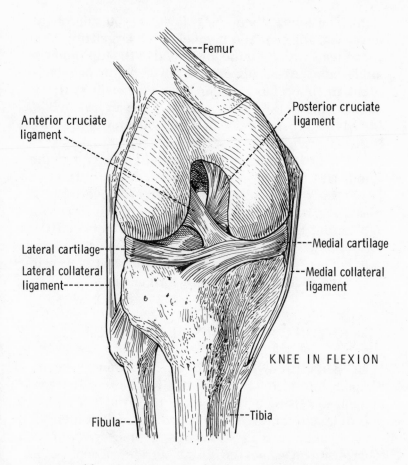

FIG. 10. *A view of your knee joint from the front, without its muscles, capsule, and kneecap. Note especially the medial and lateral collateral ligaments, the two cruciate ligaments, and the medial and lateral cartilages.*

elbow, but connects to the top of the tibia, just below and behind the latter's outside epicondyle (see illustration). The fibula, then, runs down the outside of the lower leg, adjacent and parallel to the larger tibia, and reconnects with both the lower end of the tibia and the ankle bone. At its upper and lower points of attachment, the fibula has a certain articular capability that is coordinated to the motions of the knee and the ankle, but has no direct function in the articulation of the knee itself.

The articulating surfaces at the lower end of the femur and the upper end of the tibia, where the two bones meet to form the knee joint, are covered by a glistening, rubbery, cartilage-type lining that secretes a lubricating fluid which reduces friction between the two opposed bones when they move against one another. This "articular" cartilage is *not* what we mean when we ordinarily talk about torn cartilage.

THE CARTILAGES OF THE KNEE

The cartilages we mean are two thin, crescent-shaped discs of tough tissue that are located horizontally in the space between the articulating surfaces of the tibia and femur. These two discs—called menisci, or semilunar cartilages, because of their crescent, or quarter-moon shape—cover the outside portions of the inner and outer epicondyles of the tibia where they move against the corresponding condyles of the femur, and act as cushions, or shock absorbers, for the interior of the knee joint. Since one lies in the space between the inner, or medial, aspect of the joint, and one lies on the outer, or lateral, aspect, they are referred to in medicine as medial and lateral cartilages, or menisci.

The medial and lateral cartilages (I will stick with

this term) are attached by thin bands of tissue to the edges of the inner and outer articulating condyles of the thigh and lower-leg bones which form the skeletal part of the knee joint. I will show you, a few pages ahead, how and why these cartilages become damaged. To appreciate fully what occurs, though, you should first know something about the ligaments of the knee.

THE LIGAMENTS OF THE KNEE

You have already seen that the knee is a hinge joint —it was designed by nature to move on only one plane. You have also learned that ligaments are those tissues in the body which connect bone to bone and hold the bones that form joints in proper relationship to one another. To understand the function of the principal ligaments of the knee really requires no more knowledge than this.

I did not talk at all about the ligaments that hold the elbow together because they seldom are involved in its sports-associated ailments. Because the forces on the elbow in tennis and throwing are quite different from the forces on the knee in various sports, the elbow ligaments are not usually subjected to the stresses and overloads that the knee ligaments are required to bear. It is due to the fact that the knee is a weight-bearing joint that its ligaments become so often the site and source of knee miseries.

There are four principal ligaments in the knee, two on the outside of the joint and two within. Since the two outside ligaments are the ones that are most frequently damaged, I shall start with them.

One of these ligaments is a band of tough, semi-

flexible tissue that passes vertically over the inner aspect of your knee and connects the bottom-inner end
of your thigh bone, the femur, to the top-inner end of
your primary lower-leg bone, the tibia. The connections are made along the side of the inner, or medial,
condyles of each bone. As the ligament passes over the
inner area of the joint itself it adheres to the tissue of
the medial cartilage, which is the horizontal cushion for
that side of the joint, and forms an attachment. It is
important that you keep this connection in mind, since
it is here that most knee trouble occurs.

This ligament is called the *medial collateral ligament*. It's called *medial*, as you've surely guessed by
now, because it travels over the inner aspect of the
knee joint. It's called *collateral* because it functions in
concert with another ligament. And it's called *ligament*
because it connects bone to bone. (I must confess, in its
effort to place precise designations on things, medicine
can sometimes confuse the uninitiated. But it is important that you know some of these terms, so I urge you
to press on.)

The ligament with which the medial collateral ligament works in concert is the *lateral collateral ligament*. This ligament travels over the outer aspect of the
knee joint and performs the same bone-attaching function as the inner ligament.

There are two important differences between
them, however. One is that the outer ligament connects the lower end of the femur to the fibula, the
smaller bone of the lower leg, rather than to the tibia.
This difference is important because the fibula, you'll
recall, is not part of the knee joint itself. The outer bone
of the lower leg, the fibula attaches to the tibia, the
inner bone, just below the knee joint, and at its site of

attachment, it has a slight articulation of its own. This articulation allows for the various motions in the ankle; if the articulation wasn't present just below the knee, ankle motion would be restricted. Since the outer, or lateral collateral, ligament of the knee is attached to the articulating fibula, rather than to the immobile tibia to which the inner, or medial, ligament is attached, the lateral ligament has more flexibility than the medial. As a result, it is less subject to athletic injury or damage.

The second important difference between the two collateral ligaments is that the lateral one, in passing over the outer aspect of the knee, *does not* tie in with the lateral cartilage that sits between the articulating surfaces of the joint. This cartilage is attached to the bone in the interior of the joint alone. It is less subject to tearing or other forms of damage than the medial cartilage.

Aside from connecting the thigh bone to the two lower-leg bones longitudinally and holding them together to form the knee joint, the medial and lateral collateral ligaments have a second and equally important function. They act as braces for the knee. Since the knee is designed as a hinge joint, it is not meant to move in any other than a straight back-and-forth direction. The medial and lateral collateral ligaments, then, because they are situated longitudinally along each side of the knee, prevent it from moving from side to side.

Nevertheless, many of the stresses and loads that are placed upon the knee in various sports—particularly running and contact sports—are from the side. It is under these side-stress conditions that the knee most readily gets into trouble, as we shall see in a moment. Side stresses are not the only pressures the knee must endure, however. There are also forward and backward stresses on the joint brought about by natural gravity and weight-bearing pressures on the leg. The knee joint is composed basically of the thigh bone resting on top of the main lower-leg bone. The medial and lateral collateral ligaments prevent these bones from sliding sideways against each other when various side stresses are placed on the knee. But what prevents the two bones from sliding forward and backward, one on top of the other, when forward and backward stresses are placed on the knee, say, for instance, when making a sudden stop while running?

And what about rotating stresses? We rotate our bodies when standing by using our hips. Our knees by their nature must remain straight, however. What keeps the lower ends of our femurs from unnaturally rotating on the upper ends of our tibias where they meet to form the knee joints? Although the collateral ligaments play a role, the full answer brings us to the other two primary ligaments of the knee: the *cruciate ligaments.*

The cruciate ligaments—so named because they cross each other in the form of an X—are situated within the knee joint and connect the femur to the tibia in the space between the inner and outer articulating portions of these bones. Unlike the two long collateral ligaments that travel along either side of the joint, the cruciate ligaments are short and thick. Their more exact names are the *anterior cruciate ligament* and the *posterior cruciate ligament.* The distinction between anterior and posterior is made because the former passes *in front of* the latter while diagonally crossing it to form their X-like configuration.

Because ligament connects bone to bone, one func-

tion of the two cruciate ligaments is to hold the thigh
bone and lower-leg bone together interiorly, just as the
two collateral ligaments do exteriorly. But like the exterior ligaments, they also have a bracing function; they
prevent the two knee bones from sliding back and forth
on one another and also help to inhibit the rotation of
the two bones against each other.

The *anterior* cruciate ligament crosses within the
joint from the top front of the tibia to the bottom rear
of the femur and is attached principally to these two
sites.

The *posterior* cruciate ligament originates at the
top rear of the tibia, crosses *behind* the anterior ligament without connecting to it, and attaches to the
top front portion of the femur.

The two cruciate ligaments perform in concert to
hold the knee joint together interiorly and stabilize it,
and also act with the two exterior collateral ligaments
to give the knee most of its overall rigidity. There are
still more ligaments in the knee, as well as other fibrous
bands, cords, and other parts such as its capsule, which
contribute to its basic function and stability, but these
need not concern us now. If you could visualize your
knee in all its component glory, as I can (because I have
operated on hundreds of knees), you would be con-
fronted by a veritable maze of ligaments, bones, tendons, membranes, capsules, muscles, nerves, and blood
vessels. What we are interested in here are those few
parts which, when something happens to them, can
cause trick knee to develop. Your patience and tenacity
in wading through this very important anatomy lesson
are now, I hope, about to be rewarded.

THE CAUSES OF TRICK KNEE

When speaking about the causes of the condition called trick knee, we must make the same distinction between *precipitating causes* and *underlying causes* that we made with respect to tennis elbow and will make further on in regard to other athletic ailments.

Trick knee can have a number of *precipitating causes*—injuries to the ligaments and/or cartilages brought about by a variety of severe outside blows and stresses, for instance, or lesser outside stresses which are compounded by weaknesses in the knee's supporting musculature, or spontaneous deterioration in the tissue of one or more of the knee's ligaments or cartilages. These are precipitating causes because they are events which initially cause a disorder in the knee joint.

The *underlying causes*—those causes which permit a knee damaged by injury to become a chronic trick knee—reside both in and around the knee itself, and in the psychological makeup of the sufferer. Once a cartilage (meniscus) or ligament is damaged, it cannot repair itself, as can many other tissues in our body. The reason it can't is due to the fact that cartilages and ligaments are inert tissues which receive very little nourishment from our blood-supply system. The only way they can be repaired is through surgery.

Now most of you who are saddled by trick knees undoubtedly have carried them into the present day from an earlier time when your knee was injured, from when you suffered a tear, or rupture, of one or more of your four primary knee ligaments, possibly along with one of your two cartilages. You might have been treated by a physician for the symptoms brought about by such an injury (pain, swelling, instability, etc.), but once the severe symptoms were relieved, no further medical measures were taken. Or else you might have seen your injury through on your own, without the attention of a doctor. In either case, once the pain and swelling were gone and you were able to walk without too much of a limp, you returned to your normal activities with a permanently damaged but generally serviceable knee.

It was at this point that your present-day chronic trick knee passed over from its precipitating cause to its underlying cause. From then on, the damaged tissues of your knee ligaments limited their full supporting and stabilizing functions.

But also supporting the knee, as well as being its prime movers, are the muscles that surround and attach to it. With your original injury, these muscles atrophied because you were not able to use your knee. And although your knee did eventually become serviceable again, they remained in their shrunken and weakened state. Thus your knee was partially or wholly robbed not only of the support and stability of certain ligaments but of its associated muscles as well. Consequently, your knee grew progressively weaker and less able to bear certain, even normal, stresses. It would begin to react by popping, locking, slipping, or collapsing—all full-blown signs of a trick knee.

This scenario may not have been followed exactly by your knee in arriving at its present condition, but it illustrates well how most trick-knee conditions develop and, with a possible variation or two, probably reflects accurately the evolution of your problem. Let us now take a closer look at the mechanics of trick knee.

THE MECHANICS OF TRICK KNEE

If you at one time in your life had a mild-to-severe knee injury in which a ligament and/or cartilage was torn, and you didn't have the damaged tissues repaired surgically, the likelihood is great that you now suffer from trick knee. The manner in which trick knee works can best be understood by seeing how a healthy knee works and what happens when various stresses are suddenly placed on it.

The four primary ligaments—the two collaterals and the two cruciates—are the principal supporters and stabilizers of the knee joint. The two quarter-moon-shaped, or semilunar, cartilages—one on the inner side of the joint and the other on the outer side—are its principal shock absorbers. Every time the knee joint is moved, as in walking, running, climbing stairs, and so on, these components are called upon to bear the normal stresses and shocks that occur at the joint. Let us take the stresses on the knee, and the way in which the ligaments and cartilages react to them, by steps:

1. Because the *inner*, or *medial*, collateral ligament is intended to brace the knee and prevent it from sliding or bending in an inward direction, every time a stress is applied to the knee sideways from the outside this ligament is stressed, as is the horizontally situated medial meniscus, or cartilage, to which it is fused. Such a stress is called a *valgus stress*.

2. Because the *outer*, or *lateral*, collateral ligament is intended to brace the knee and prevent it from sliding or bending in an outward direction, every time a stress is applied to the

knee sideways from the inside this ligament is
stressed. Such a stress is called a *varus stress*.
The horizontally situated lateral cartilage,
however, is not stressed because it is not attached to, and does not tie in with, the lateral
ligament; it will be stressed, though, if the lateral ligament cannot wholly absorb the force
applied against the knee.

3. Because the *anterior cruciate* ligament within
the knee joint is intended to brace the knee
and prevent both the femur from sliding backward on the tibia and hyperextension of the
knee (extension beyond the normal straight-
leg position), every time a stress is applied to
the knee from *the front and above* or from
behind and below, this ligament is stressed.

4. Because the *posterior cruciate* ligament within
the knee joint is intended to brace the knee
and prevent both the femur from sliding forward on the tibia and hyperextension of the
knee, every time a stress is applied to the knee
from the *front and below* or from *behind and
above,* this ligament is stressed.

5. Because all four ligaments are intended to
brace the knee and help prevent the two
bones of its joint from rotating one upon the
other, every time a rotatory stress is applied to
the knee from any direction, such as when piv-
oting, all four will be stressed, some more than
others, depending on the direction and force
of the stress. Furthermore, the two horizontal
cartilages in the inner and outer portions of
the joint will also be stressed, since the forces
of rotation act directly upon them.

I have put these steps in series and have stated
them in the form of axioms because they describe the

principal forces that act upon the knee during its normal activity and especially during athletic activities. Now there remains one final axiom to be stated:

6. During all athletic activities the knee is hardly ever restricted to just one of the foregoing stresses at a time; rather it is subject to all these stresses in varying combinations of force and intensity.

We all learned in our high-school physics classes that for every force there is a counterforce, for every action there is a reaction. This phenomenon is as basic to nature as apples are to apple pie. Unfortunately, the human knee has never learned this law, and its failure to do so is at the root of the trouble it gets itself into. Yet the knee itself can't be blamed. Nor can nature. We must blame ourselves—for by popularizing the sports we've invented to amuse ourselves, we have placed demands on the structures of our knees, particularly their ligaments and cartilages, that nature had no way of anticipating when she designed them.

The ligaments and cartilages of the knee were designed for what we might call the normal functions of our legs: to propel us from one place to another. Normal locomotion never required the knee to do anything more than to bend rearward (flex) and straighten out (extend). But the advent of certain sports—football, baseball, tennis, basketball, skiing, skating, and the like —demanded a whole new collection of functions for the knee that the knee just did not have time in its evolution to fulfill. These functions required the knee to withstand forces it was not engineered to withstand, and the result has been a veritable epidemic of damaged or trick knees.

The most common form of damage comes from an excessive force—either from a blow or through an overstress caused by a sudden shifting of weight— against the healthy knee from its outer, or lateral, side. The force can be *directly* from the side or *diagonally* from the side. No matter the precise compass point from which it comes, if its power is in excess of the knee's ability to withstand it, damage to one or more ligaments and cartilages will occur.*

When an excessive and sudden outside-to-inside force is applied to the knee, the knee is put under pressure to rotate and bend inward unnaturally. The medial collateral ligament, in its effort to prevent the knee from so bending, is stretched beyond its normal flexibility. As a result, fibers in the ligament begin to tear or separate from one another. Depending on the amount of the force, only a few fibers will tear, many fibers will tear, or all the fibers will tear, leading to a complete rupture of the ligament. With the ligament partially or completely torn, it loses part or all of its medial bracing function, and the knee is free to bend inward.

In addition, when the medial ligament is excessively stretched, and thereby torn, it is liable to take the medial cartilage—the flat, semilunar disc which is set horizontally into the joint itself as a shock absorber— with it. That is, because this cartilage is attached to the ligament, an excessive stretching of the ligament pulls on the cartilage, causing fibers in the cartilage to tear as well.

When the excessive and sudden outside-to-inside

---

*No two healthy knees are the same. Some are naturally "tighter," others naturally "looser." One knee can withstand a force under which another will collapse. But every knee has its collapsing point. Count yourself lucky if you have naturally hardy knees.

force is not directly from the side but is applied diagonally—either forward or rearward of the knee—the
same sequence of events occurs. But in these cases the
cruciate ligaments become involved as well.

A diagonal blow or force from the front quarter
will not only pressure the knee to bend inward, it will
also—depending on whether it is applied above or below the knee—pressure the femur, or thigh bone, to
slide backward or forward over the tibia at the joint.
The same force applied diagonally from the rear quarter will exert similar pressures, again depending on
whether applied above or below the knee.

Thus, the anterior cruciate ligament will also often
tear along with the medial collateral ligament and cartilage. When it does, the knee joint ends up with a
double instability: it is unstable in a sideways direction,
and it is unstable in a forward direction.

These are the most common injuries of the knee.
Injuries to the lateral collateral ligament are rarer,
mainly for two reasons. One is, as I have noted, that
sudden and excessive inside-to-outside forces on the
knee do not occur with anywhere near the frequency
of outside-to-inside forces. Thus, the knee is seldom
pressured to bend outward. The second reason is that
even when the knee *is* pressured to bend outward, its
outer brace, the lateral collateral ligament, is given
help in withstanding the pressure by another tough
band of tissue which I haven't mentioned yet. This is a
wide fibrous band that stretches longitudinally over the
side of the knee from the femur to the tibia, covering
the lateral ligament and providing the knee with extra
lateral support. It is called the *iliotibial band.*

If you will stand up with both your legs straight and
your feet slightly apart and flat on the floor, you'll see

what I mean when I say that the inner, or medial, aspects of your knees are much more vulnerable to injury than the outer, or lateral, aspects. If you try to press your knees outward you'll find that you encounter a good deal more resistance than when you press them inward. This is primarily because of the extra lateral support provided by the iliotibial tract.

This, then, is the basic mechanics of injuries to the principal supporting ligaments of the knee. An excessive force applied to the knee in an outside-to-inside direction—either directly sideways or diagonally— causes the bracing ligaments along the inside of the knee and often within the knee joint itself to tear, or rupture. The immediate results of such injuries is pain, swelling, and joint instability. Once the pain and swelling have abated, the joint instability remains if the damaged ligaments are not repaired surgically. And it is made even more unstable by the atrophying and weakening of the muscles around the knee which would otherwise add to its support.

If you understand the mechanics of such knee injury, then you will understand the mechanics of trick knee. For trick knee is basically nothing more than a knee which has been made unstable by torn ligaments and cartilage.

The two primary manifestations of trick knee are the unexpected "collapse" of the knee, usually when you are changing direction while walking or running, and the unexpected "locking" of the knee in any number of positions it might find itself in. If you have a trick knee, it will certainly display one of these manifestations and will often display both.

A trick knee does not really "collapse," however; it only appears to. What happens is fundamentally the same as what occurs when an excessive force is applied to a healthy and stable knee: the medial cartilage, the medial collateral ligament, and sometimes one or both of the cruciate ligaments are stretched beyond their limits. They tear, or rupture, compromising the knee's normal stability and causing it to bend in unnatural directions.

But in the case of trick knee, this stability has already been compromised. One or more ligaments had been torn at some earlier time—probably the cartilage too—so that much of the knee's inward stability, and perhaps some of its forward-backward stability, has been lost. With this lost stability, *even less than normal* forces applied to the knee in a straight or diagonal outside-inside direction will cause the knee to bend inward or slide back and forth. Such inward bending or back-and-forth sliding is similar to what occurs when an *excessive* force is applied—the knee is forced to bend and/or slide unnaturally. With the affected ligaments already loosened by unrepaired tears, or ruptures, they are unable to brace against these motions, and the knee bends or slides further until all vertical stability is lost and it "gives way."

Unless caught in time, the "collapsing" version of trick knee will usually sustain additional injuries and tears in the already damaged ligaments and cartilage, thereby creating swelling, pain, and further instability. So the knee becomes progressively more weak with each episode, until eventually the victim is required to wear a brace or to have the knee repaired surgically.

In the "locking" version, which is the more frequent manifestation of trick knee, the knee will not necessarily become more weak although the pain and "strange" sensation of "locking" will be just as infuriating. The locking of the knee is not really a locking at all. It is more of a temporary displacement in the normal relationship between the components of the knee joint brought about by one or two of several possible causes. These causes, of course, have to do with the loss of directional stability which is caused by damaged ligaments and cartilage.

Locking generally expresses itself in four slightly different sensations: (1) The knee feels as though it has slipped laterally, with the outer portion "locked." (2) The knee feels as though it has slipped forward, with the front portion locked. (3) The knee feels as though it has slipped backwards, with the rear portion locked. (4) The knee does not feel as though it has slipped in any particular direction, but simply becomes locked in its normal straight flexion-extension function. The more common of these locking sensations are the first and the fourth, and an explanation of them will help you understand the other two.

As to the first, the most frequent of all knee-ligament damage occurs, as I have said, in the medial collateral ligament, that ligament whose primary support function is to prevent abnormal inward bending of the knee. It also helps, along with the cruciate ligaments, to keep the knee joint itself from sliding in a sideways direction and thus displacing, even slightly, the articulating surfaces of the two leg bones that form the joint. When the medial collateral ligament is damaged, it becomes flaccid rather than taut, thus losing its ability to fulfill wholly its bracing function. It not only allows inward "give" of the joint, it also permits a slight or even considerable displacement of the bone surfaces. It is this displacement that creates the locking sensation. It also creates a greater stress on other intact structures.

Lateral displacement comes about when unequal lateral pressures or stresses are applied to the leg above and below the weakened knee. In other words, if a lateral force is applied to the leg below the knee, the knee joint will tend to open on the inside due to the reduced support of the flaccid medial collateral ligament. This medial opening causes a "popping" sensation, and if the bones of the joint are displaced sufficiently, they can become "locked." Finding themselves out of their proper alignment, they will be unable to articulate properly one against the other.

Many individuals with trick knee—especially men —complain that their knees tend to pop or lock when they are simply sitting in that traditional way American men have of sitting: with one lower leg crossed laterally over the opposite thigh. In this position, the outside part of the lower leg, just above the ankle, rests on the top of the opposite knee. Unbeknownst to those who sit this way, their lower leg bones are being pushed upwards (that is, inwards) as the weight of their crossed leg rests horizontally on its opposite. The thigh of the crossed leg, which is also raised in a horizontal position, has no separate support for its weight, so it tends to follow the law of gravity, to fall toward the floor (that is, outward).

Hence, while the thigh of the crossed leg seeks to go downward (outward) through the force of gravity, the lower part of the leg is held in check. This, in effect, creates a counterforce, pressing the lower leg upward (inward). When the man is the owner of a ruptured medial collateral ligament, and possibly of a compromised anterior cruciate ligament, his knee will tend to slide laterally and even rotate slightly, causing the inner components of his joint to displace. This motion will, in turn, produce the familiar popping or locking sensation.

Women experience a similar phenomenon, and it derives from their special way of sitting—with the back of one knee crossed over the top of the other, the familiar "legs-crossed" position. Here the force is on the back of the crossed leg, just below the knee joint, and it is a force that pushes the top of the tibia forward. If the woman has damaged ligaments—particularly an anterior cruciate ligament—her tibia will be forced forward against her stationary thigh bone. The resulting displacement of articulating components within the joint will cause a locking sensation.

The other manifestation of locking—the fourth in my description of a page or so ago—involves one or both of the menisci, or cartilages, of the knee. You will recall, again, that I have described these cartilages as being situated horizontally in the space between the articulating knobs of the joint. They both act as cushions, particularly around the outer portions of the knobs, and also aid in keeping the lower and upper knobs in proper alignment. The medial cartilage is torn ten times more frequently than the lateral cartilage because it is less mobile as a result of its attachment to the medial collateral ligament. When the medial collateral ligament is ruptured or otherwise damaged, the medial cartilage is usually damaged as well. So it is the inner cartilage (or medial meniscus) that is most often the villain in this type of locking.

What happens is that when the medial collateral ligament is overstressed, it pulls at the medial cartilage so that both are torn or ruptured. Because the damaged cartilage is actually set into the joint, a partially separated portion of it can float free within. When the knee is being used, this piece occasionally becomes lodged between the two articulating surfaces. When this occurs, the natural flexion-extension motion of the joint is disturbed, and the joint locks. In other words, the articulating surfaces of the joint are blocked by the intruding piece of stray cartilage.

UNLOCKING A LOCKED KNEE

What to do when your knee locks? The trick-knee veteran can usually feel a lock coming on, and this is why I have used the term "sensation" to describe the phenomenon. The sensation is hard to describe, but is familiar to all victims of such knee problems; it is akin to a feeling that the interior of the knee is being pressed outward from within in all directions, as though a bubble is expanding and about to burst. At just the moment of "bursting," the knee will either "pop" and go back to normal, or it will "lock." As the "pop" occurs the individual with quick reflexes will be able to adjust the position of his knee to prevent it from locking. The slower-reflexed person might not be able to act in time, and knee-lock will result.

The usual manner of "unlocking" a locked knee is to flex or extend it abruptly, or shake it violently, withstanding the intense temporary pain for the sake of restoring it to normal. I am sure that all of you with trick knee have your favorite, time-tested methods. Some newcomers to trick knee are inclined to panic, however, and can end up in worse shape than when they started. They go into contortions that can cause further damage to the joint and even broken bones.

The best principle to follow, as an emergency procedure when your knee locks in a sideways or front-

or-back position, is to remember that its articulating surfaces have been displaced laterally, or to the fore or rear. This means that a force—even if only the force of weight and gravity—has displaced your lower-leg bone (tibia) in relation to your thigh bone (femur), or vice versa. Your job is to reverse that force so that *dis*placement becomes *re*placement. This can either be done manually or by simply reversing the forces of weight and gravity.*

The latter is usually the quickest and easiest. Generally, all one need do is to suspend the affected leg in the direction opposite to the locked position. For instance, if your knee locks laterally to the outside, it is usually because the weight of the thigh and the force of gravity have forced your thigh bone laterally and to the outside of your lower-leg bone. By suspending your leg in a semihorizontal position so that the weight of the thigh bone falls downward or inward, the knee joint will slip back into proper alignment.

In the case of a rarer forward knee-lock, the thigh bone has slid forward over your lower-leg bone. You can usually correct this by slowly raising your leg in a kicking motion: the weight-and-gravity factor will encourage your thigh bone to slip back into its proper position. Forward knee-lock generally occurs during extreme flexing or bending of the knee, as in squatting maneuvers. If you find yourself suddenly on the floor or ground with your knee locked in such a manner, it is best to turn onto your back and then kick your leg into the air.

Rear knee-lock is mostly associated with hyperex-

---

*Knee displacement is not the same as dislocation of the knee. Dislocation of the knee sometimes refers to dislocation of the kneecap, which I will discuss further along in this chapter. But true knee dislocation falls under the category of injury and is beyond the scope of this book.

tension; in other words, in straightening your leg out, the thigh bone slides rearward over your lower-leg bone, and your knee becomes locked in the straight position. Here the object is to use the forces of weight and gravity to move the thigh bone forward again, and this can be best achieved by raising your straightened leg behind you in a reverse-kicking motion.

If these measures don't work, manual adjustment is called for. This consists mainly of forcing the recalcitrant bones back into their proper relationship. Thus, with lateral lock, by pressing the outside of your thigh inward with one hand, and the inside of your lower leg outward with the other, you should be able to move your knee out of its lock. Don't, however, try to do this with your weight on your leg, for the pressure of your weight will only make it more difficult and cause further pain. Suspend your leg so that your foot is off the ground, and let gravity help you.

The real secret of unlocking your knee is the ability to relax. The reason it locks in the first place is because its already weakened supporting ligaments and muscles have become fatigued. The muscles go into spasm, holding the knee in its locked position, and the spasms are compounded by the fact that you tense all the muscles in your leg while frantically trying to relieve the lock. Your best bet is to try to relax your leg muscles because often, as the muscles relax, the knee will slip out of the lock of its own accord.

Of course, if a lock cannot be immediately relieved, you should then seek medical help. It is not advisable, except under emergency circumstances, to let a friend or passerby attempt to unlock your knee. More often than not, because the good samaritan has no idea of how your lock "feels," he or she will inadvertently cause more serious damage.

YOUR LIGAMENTS: TORN OR RUPTURED?

Here we come to another element of confusion among knee victims: what constitutes a *torn* ligament or cartilage and what a *ruptured* ligament or cartilage? Indeed, what is the difference between "torn" and "ruptured," and how do the two categories affect knee function? To understand this is to go a long way toward understanding the treatment and cure of trick knee.

The ligaments of the body, as I have described, are comprised of countless tiny strands of fiber layered and woven together into a tough, semielastic tissue. There are more than a hundred of these items in the body, and their main functions are to connect bone to bone, to act as checkreins so that the bones they connect cannot be thrown out of alignment, and to serve as braces for the joints. When excessive forces are placed on them they become damaged and lose their ability to perform fully their checkrein and bracing functions. The elasticity of ligament tissue is far from infinite, and when it is stretched beyond its capacity, something's got to give. What gives are the fibers that compose the tissue: when they are stretched beyond their capacity, they simply pull apart.

A simple example of this is when you pull on both ends of a short string. If you pull hard enough, the outer strands will begin to separate. Harder still, and the string will snap apart. So, too, a ligament (although some ligaments can withstand greater stretching forces than others). When a ligament is stretched beyond its capacity, some of its fibrous strands will pull apart. When it is stretched *far* beyond its capacity, all the strands that hold it together will separate. It will not snap completely apart, as a string, but the effect will be the same—it will lose its tautness and become lax, no longer able to fulfill its supporting and bracing functions.

Now, many patients I see who have knee-ligament problems seem to think that there is some sort of quantitative difference between a torn ligament and a ruptured ligament; that is, they labor under the misconception that a torn ligament is somehow not as serious or disabling as a ruptured one. Again, this is probably partly the fault of us doctors, who sometimes are a bit careless with our semantics. But it is also the fault of the press—especially sportswriters and announcers—who are prone to make distinctions between torn and ruptured ligaments when describing the knee ailments of our popular athletic heroes. By so doing they have succeeded in leaving the impression in the awareness of the general public that a torn ligament is different from a ruptured ligament.

The fact is that a torn ligament is the same as a ruptured one. It is not the adjective which determines the severity of a ligament injury, it is the nature of the injury itself. If only a few strands of fiber in an individual's knee ligament are pulled apart, the condition might be described as a partial tear or rupture. With this situation, the ligament loses *some* of its bracing-and-supportive capability, but not all. It follows that the more strands that are pulled apart, the less the ligament will be able to perform its function, and the more unstable the knee joint will be. It is this inability to perform up to full capability on the part of the ligament (and cartilage) that produces trick knee.

A complete tear or rupture means that *all* the strands in the ligament have been pulled apart. The ligament is totally lax and provides *no* stability or support at all. When this occurs, the only way stability can be restored is through surgery. Without surgery, the victim will not only have a trick knee, he will have difficulty walking in any kind of normal manner and will be unable to participate in any sport.

Therefore, surgery is a prerequisite to the cure of a totally unstable knee. It also provides the definitive cure for trick knee. However, many trick-knee victims —particularly those whose knees are only occasionally bothersome—prefer to avoid surgery and try to "live with" their condition. To do so successfully, they must turn to the "management" of their knees.

TRICK KNEE: SURGERY OR MANAGEMENT?

A totally torn, or ruptured, ligament should be repaired surgically as soon as possible because the earlier the repair, the better are the chances of restoration of full knee junction. Surgery consists of opening up the knee in the area of the rupture, attempting to suture together the torn ends, and if that is not possible, to reconstruct a reasonable facsimile out of other tissue, such as the iliotibial band or an expendable tendon. Care is taken that proper tension is restored to the ligament so that once the tissue transplant "takes," the repaired ligament will be able to fulfill its bracing and supportive function again. Then the incision is closed up and the leg is placed in a cast so that the everything will have a chance to heal. After the cast is removed, the patient must go through a period of physical therapy and intensive leg exercise to restore full knee motion and muscular support. If these aspects of recuperation are successfully concluded, the ligament will be almost as good as new.

This is the fundamental process of knee-ligament surgery, although it may entail additional surgical procedures such as the removal of torn cartilage and the resectioning of other tissues in the knee to give the repaired ligament further support. Surgery for trick knee follows approximately the same course and, if performed properly and early, is almost certain to overcome the condition.

Much that goes into a decision as to whether or not to operate depends on the psychological attitude of the trick-knee victim. Medically speaking, the operation is not life-saving. But for the patient, it often is. Chances are that eventually a person with a torn medial collateral ligament or a torn cartilage, or both, will require surgery. If the difficulty is just an isolated anterior cruciate ligament, however, the likelihood is that the person will be able to get along without surgery.

More seriously victimized trick-knee patients, on the other hand, may absolutely require an operation—again, medically speaking—in order to function normally, but will resist the idea with all their might because they are psychologically unprepared to face the terrors they imagine such surgery entails. Although the only terrors are a certain amount of temporary postoperative pain and discomfort, they would rather endure the permanent pain and debility in their knees than the temporary pain and discomfort.

You can see, then, that the whole question of surgery on a partially damaged knee is, if you will overlook a bad pun, a tricky one. I am certainly not going to recommend that if you have a trick knee you should immediately consider surgery to correct it. I can only recommend that you consult a physician qualified to deal with knee problems and, based on his diagnosis, prognosis, and recommendations, arrive at your own enlightened decision. I can assure you, however, that if your knee significantly hinders your pleasure in athletic endeavors, or even your enjoyment of daily life, the appropriate knee surgery has an excellent chance of reversing these factors.

Medical diagnosis is, of course, the key to any decision about the kind of treatment you should receive. When you consult a doctor about a trick-knee complaint he will base his diagnosis on three general procedures. The first of these is your medical history, especially that part of it which relates to your knee and its symptoms. A complete history of your knee—its past injuries, its frequency of pain and malfunction, and other symptoms—is very important in giving the physician a clear picture of what *may* be wrong with it.

The second procedure will be a general physical examination followed by a specific examination of your knee. The doctor will sit or lay you down and then, with his arms and hands, apply various opposing forces to your knee to see in which directions it reveals instability and looseness. He will also evaluate the relative strength and weakness of your muscles. From these tests he can get an accurate idea about which of the vital support-brace components of your knee are damaged, and the extent to which they are damaged.

The third procedure will be a series of X rays of your knee taken from different angles so that all the components of the joint can be seen. If the doctor suspects cartilage damage within the joint, he will also order an *arthrogram*, an X ray taken with a special fluid injected with air into the joint, which coats the cartilage and reveals the site and extent of damage.

Based on his findings, the physician will formulate

a prognosis for your knee without surgery. A prognosis is nothing more than a medical prediction, founded on the physician's experience and knowledge, of how the knee will function in the future either with or without surgical repair. If he concludes that the knee is not damaged seriously enough to require immediate surgery, he will provide you with a "management" program under which you can strengthen the knee's supporting muscles and thereby reduce the stresses which the damaged components are presently required to bear. Such a program consists mostly of leg exercises, a few of which I will describe a few pages further on. In many cases, the faithful implementation of this program will actually reduce the incidence of trick knee and will enable you to continue to engage in your favorite sport without the constant fear of your knee collapsing or locking. However, I should point out that you still have damaged components in your knee, and that further severe stresses on these components may well compound the damage, eventually requiring you to undergo surgery if you wish to continue with athletics.

If the physician's prognosis is less optimistic, and he feels that your knee will continue to grow worse despite the management program, he will advise you either to give up your sports activities altogether or submit your knee to surgical repair. This is when you will find yourself faced with a hard decision. If you are like most weekend athletes I have treated, you will at first resist an operation and continue to struggle along in your sport (for after all, none of us likes to think of ourselves as vincible). But the likelihood is great that sooner or later you will end up on the operating table. And all it will usually take is one further episode of knee collapse while you are racing to retrieve a cross-court backhand or zigging out for a sideline pass.

Again, rest assured that if ligament and/or cartilage surgery is necessary, the chances of it being completely successful are very bright. It is a routine operation among orthopedists these days, and except for some postoperative knee pain, you have little to fear. And whatever pain and recuperative discipline are required are more than offset by the potential rewards— the ability to pursue your athletic interests without pain and without physical debility.

One other factor that makes surgery desirable is its ability to head off further knee-joint complications before they have a chance to develop. Remember that if any of your knee ligaments or cartilages are damaged, your knee will be required to operate in an abnormal, even if still serviceable, manner. That is, the motion and articulation within the joint will not be as smooth as nature designed. Abnormal or out-of-alignment joint articulation will often, over a long period, cause excessive and abnormal wear on the joint's surfaces. This can lead not only to a breakdown of other supporting and bracing components of the knee, but also to arthritis in the joint itself as the worn surfaces become inflamed. And I'm sure I don't have to tell you that arthritis is considerably more painful and incapacitating than trick knee.

MANAGING A TRICK KNEE
WITHOUT SURGERY

If your doctor believes that you can get along without surgery and that by faithfully implementing a management program you have a good chance of overcoming your trick knee, he will prescribe a series of leg exercises designed to strengthen the extensor and flexor muscles that both move the knee and serve to provide it with support. In discussing these muscles, we come to the second important component in knee function.

You'll recall how I described the elbow joint as being provided with its flexion-extension mobility by groups of muscles in the forearm which attach to the bone of the upper arm, and by groups of muscles in the upper arm which attach to the two bones of the forearm. The knee works on the same principle, as do all the joints of the body: if muscles from one side of the joint did not cross the joint and attach to the other side, the joint could not be moved.

There are three important muscles around the knee that provide it primarily with motion and secondarily with support. These are:

1. The *Quadriceps*, or primary knee-extensor muscles, along the front of the thigh;
2. The *Hamstrings*, or primary knee-flexor muscles, along the back of the thigh
3. The *Gastrocnemii*, or secondary knee-flexor muscles, along the back and sides of the calf. The gastrocnemius also enables you to lift your heel off the ground, as I shall explain in a later chapter.

The *quadriceps* is the most vital of all the knee muscles—mainly because it is the knee's only extensor muscle, and because extension is required to enable us to stand on our feet, let alone walk. The quadriceps is not just one muscle, though. It gets its name from the fact that it is formed by four (quad) interrelated muscles which run along the front of the thighbone and blend

into one conjoined tendon that inserts into the kneecap.

Now—before I continue with the muscles—I must
call a time-out so that I can describe the function of the
kneecap, for here is a third vital component in knee
function.

The kneecap (properly called the *patella*) is a separate bone of the knee. It is a flat, oval-shaped structure;
it is situated directly in front of the knee joint and was
evidently designed to protect the joint back in the days
when man crawled around on his hands and knees.*

But this was, and is, not its only function. Because
the joint is mobile, the kneecap cannot be connected
directly to both bones of the joint; it must be free to
move in response to the motion of the joint. It possesses
this freedom by being attached to only one bone, the
tibia, or lower-leg bone. But even then it is not *directly*
attached, because it needs to be able to move when the
joint is flexed. So the attachment is made through the
medium of a long, wide ligament called the *patellar
ligament* (remember, again, that ligament connects
bone to bone).

That takes care of its attachment to the leg below
the knee. But how is it attached above? Many of you
would probably guess, using simple logic, that it is connected to the bone of the thigh immediately above the
knee. The logic is foolproof. However, in this case it
deceives because the kneecap is not attached to the
thigh bone. Instead, it is attached to the quadriceps
muscle by the *quadriceps tendon.*

---

*Support for this theory is evidenced by the fact that we have bones similar
to the kneecap protecting the palm joints of our fingers and thumbs, and also
protecting the undersides of our large toe joint. These bones serve no other
purpose than to protect the joints from weight-bearing shocks.

This leads us to the third vital role the kneecap plays in the function of the knee. I said before that the flexor and extensor muscles pass over the joints and attach to the bones on the opposite sides. Here again the logic is impeccable. And here again it deceives, for the quadriceps muscle of the knee is an exception to the rule. Rather than passing over the knee and inserting into the tibia below, the quadriceps attaches to the kneecap, which in turn attaches to the tibia below through the patellar ligament. So the kneecap is the substitute for the quadriceps being attached directly to the other side of the joint.

More about this later, when we come to ailments around the kneecap itself. Let me return now to the muscles that give the knee its motion and support, and describe how these muscles can be strengthened to counteract the weaknesses which cause trick knee.

Returning to the quadriceps muscles, this group acts to extend or straighten the knee. When they are contracted they pull on the kneecap. The force and power of their contraction is transmitted through the kneecap to the tibia, and the leg is pulled up and held straight.

You can easily feel your quadriceps, or knee extensors. They are the thick muscles, just above your knee, which extend up the front of your thigh. Notice how they seem to "bunch" when you extend your leg and how the contracting force runs all the way up your thigh to your hips. Now feel just below your knee for the small, but prominent, protuberance on the front of your shin. This is called the *anterior tibial tubercle* and is the site at which your patellar ligament attaches your kneecap, and therefore your quadriceps muscles, to your tibia. It is the flow of extensor power through your

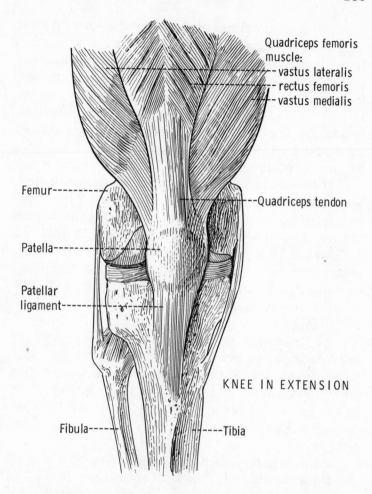

Quadriceps femoris
muscle:
-- vastus lateralis
-- rectus femoris
-- vastus medialis

Femur--------
Quadriceps tendon

Patella--------

Patellar
ligament--------

KNEE IN EXTENSION

Fibula----- -----Tibia

FIG. 11. *Another front view of your knee joint,*
this time showing the patella (kneecap), the compo-
nents of the quadriceps *muscle, the* quadriceps
tendon, and the patellar ligament.

kneecap and its ligament to the tibia that gives the knee
its extensor effect.

The primary flexor muscles of the knee are the hamstring group, which run down the back of the thigh from the pelvis. Again, like the quadriceps, this is not a single muscle but a series of interwoven and interacting muscles. Unlike the quadriceps, however, they attach directly to the lower leg bones just below, behind, and to the side of the knee. When they are contracted they pull on the top rear portions of the lower leg, causing it to raise and the knee to flex or bend.

The secondary flexor muscles—the *gastrocnemii*—are situated along the back of the lower leg. They originate from two heads at the lower rear of the thigh bone, then continue down behind the knee and through the calf, where they join with another muscle called the *soleus* to form the bulge of the calf. These muscles terminate in the heel, being attached thereto by the Achilles tendon, and act in concert with the hamstrings of the thigh to bring about full flexion of the knee.

All three of these muscle groups, besides producing extension and flexion, also provide secondary support for the knee. Since most ligament damage occurs when the knee is slightly bent, with the weight of the body upon it, the extensor, or quadriceps, muscles are those that figure most importantly in the joint's structural stability.

I wrote earlier in these pages about how often I observe a direct correlation between cases of trick knee and weak quadriceps muscles. The direct cause of trick knee is one or more partially torn or otherwise damaged ligaments and cartilage. An indirect cause is weakness and atrophy of the quadriceps muscles, a condition that is usually a by-product of the knee injuries which, when uncorrected surgically, permit trick knee to develop.

As we know, when one or more knee ligaments are damaged, they cannot be restored except through surgery. When quadriceps weakness ensues as a result of such damage, however, strength can be restored without surgical intervention. When the quadriceps muscles are permitted to remain weak and flabby, they contribute to the instability of the knee when it is in extension. And when all these conditions exist, episodes of trick knee are likely to occur.

By restoring and strengthening his or her quadriceps muscles, the trick-knee victim encourages these muscles to take up some of the slack caused by the damaged ligaments and to provide the ligaments with much-needed help in trying to keep the knee stable in spite of their defects. Thus, it becomes imperative for trick-knee sufferers who decide against surgery to commit themselves to the restoration of their quadriceps, indeed, to restoring them even beyond their strength prior to the original damage. This is best achieved through the following leg exercises:

Exercise 1. Quadriceps Extensor Raise
Sit on a high platform so that the backs of your thighs rest on the surface and your knees and lower legs hang over the side without touching the floor. Keep your back straight and cross your arms over your chest to avoid giving the leg you'll be exercising any help. Then, keeping your thigh solidly pressed to the platform, slowly extend or raise your lower leg until your leg is straight and horizontal. Hold for a count of five, then return your leg to the starting position.

Repeat this exercise thirty times, or as many times as you can. As the strain begins to tell *do not* start to swing your upper body back and forth to give your leg a start. When you can do the leg-raise thirty times without fatigue, it is time to add weight. Purchase adjustable ankle weights. (These are bands that strap around your ankles and have pockets in which two-pound lead weights are inserted; they are available in any sports-supply store.)

Start with two pounds and work up again to a comfortable thirty repetitions. When you can achieve this, add another two pounds, and so on up. When you can finally raise your lower leg thirty consecutive times with a total weight equal to ten percent of your body weight, you will know that your quadriceps muscles have reached an ideal strength—ideal, that is, for a healthy knee. But you're knee isn't healthy, so you have a way to go yet.

Continue to add weight in two-pound increments until you are capable of performing thirty repetitions at a weight that is the equivalent of at least 15 percent of your body weight. Thus, if you weigh 120 pounds and can achieve thirty repetitions at eighteen pounds of ankle weight, your quadriceps are now sufficiently strong to do some of the job of your damaged ligaments. The same is true if you weigh 200 pounds and can lift thirty pounds of weight thirty consecutive times. You should do this exercise at least once a day until you have reached the ideal level (don't be afraid to go beyond the ideal level). Thereafter, you should continue to do it at least twice a week to maintain the strength of your quadriceps.

One point worth mentioning here is that it is advisable to work on the quadriceps of your other knee as well. Some of you may have weak second knees in addition to your trick knee without being aware of it. By working on the second knee in this and subsequent exercises, you can only help yourself by preventing the potential development of a second trick knee.

Exercise 2.   Straight Leg Raise
Lie flat on your back on the floor with both legs fully extended. (If you have a bad back, extend only the leg you'll be exercising while keeping your other leg bent with your foot flat on the floor.) Stiffen your exercising leg and slowly raise it until it reaches a forty-five-degree angle to the floor. Hold it there for a count of five, then return it slowly to the floor. Repeat until you can do forty repetitions comfortably. Then begin adding your ankle weights in two pound increments.

Whereas Exercise 1 strengthens the quadriceps muscles directly above the knee, this exercise will strengthen these muscles all the way up your thigh to your hip, adding to the knee's upright stability.

Exercise 3.   Straight Leg Abductor
This is similar to Exercise 2, except here you lie on your side and abduct, or raise, your stiffened leg sideways as high from the floor as you can, holding it each time for a count of five. Use the same repetition-weight increases.

Exercise 4.   Knee Rotation
This is a simple isometric exercise intended to strengthen all the muscles that pass around your knee, lend it support, and prevent it from rotating abnormally. Simply sit on a chair with your knees bent and your feet on the floor. (You might sit at a table so that you can grasp its sides for support.) Put your feet together, and then press your toes toward each other,

holding them together for a count of five with as much force as you can muster. Then relax and repeat for twenty repetitions.

Follow this up with the very same routine applied to your heels. This toe-and-heel exercise can be performed anywhere and should be done at least three times a day.

These exercises won't cure your trick knee, but if they are faithfully executed over a period of time they will certainly enable you to manage your problem successfully and continue with your favorite sports. Of course, you should try to avoid sudden shifts in direction on your weak knee, but otherwise you should feel free to engage in any activity with full gusto.

JUMPER'S KNEE

Here is an ailment that is the bane of recreational basketball and volleyball enthusiasts. Indeed, it even strikes *professional* basketball players. Basketball fans will remember a few years ago when Willis Reed, the captain and star center of the New York Knicks, was out of action for half the season, then valiantly tried to come back and lead his team in the championship playoffs against the Los Angeles Lakers. He failed to get very far, although his brief presence seemed to inspire his teammates. Reed's problem was a bad case of jumper's knee, or what is called in medical circles *patellar tendinitis.*

Patellar tendinitis is an extremely painful inflammation of the patellar tendon just above the kneecap. By now you should be fairly knowledgeable about the anatomy of the knee (although I have yet to cover the joint in all its numerous aspects). You will recall from my discussion a few pages back that the kneecap, or patella, has several functions, and that one of them is to act as a connection between the extensor quadriceps muscles at the front of the thigh just above the knee and the tibia, or lower-leg bone, just below the knee. It is the architecture of this connection that allows the knee both to extend and flex as easily as it does.

In a sense, the kneecap is to the knee what the lateral epicondyle is to the elbow: it provides the joint with its fulcrum effect. But in so doing, it is subject to the very same difficulties that produce tennis elbow—which, you'll remember, is an inflammation of the extensor tendon that connects the elbow's forearm extensor muscles to the upper portion of the elbow joint itself.

The patellar tendon in the knee—the tendon that attaches the knee's extensor thigh muscles to the kneecap—is an extensor tendon. Every time you extend your knee—in walking, running, and the like—the patellar tendon comes into play. And as with tennis elbow, every time an excessive force, stress, or shock is applied to the tendon, it will tend to stretch and tear.

It is because such stresses are applied during jumping movements that patellar tendinitis is known as jumper's knee. And one need only look at the mechanics of jumping to understand how and why it develops—especially in basketball and volleyball players. In these sports, the jump is a fundamental maneuver. Such jumping is generally a vertical movement, as opposed to the type of jump in which one leaves the ground at one spot and lands in another, two or three feet distant. It is the vertical characteristic of the basketball or volleyball jump that causes most of the problems that result in patellar tendinitis.

The basketball or volleyball jump requires you first to flex your knees in order to give your legs the coil-spring power needed for optimum height, and then to extend your knees abruptly as you leave the ground. This sudden flexion-to-extension places a tremendous load on your knee's extensor muscles, the quadriceps, and on the tendon that connects them to your knee, the patellar tendon, which results in a tendency to hyper-extend. Multiply this tendency by the 50 or 100 jumps you might make in a basketball or volleyball game, and you'll see how repeatedly your patellar tendon is strained.

Now the patellar tendon is, as I have indicated, strong, tough, and elastic to a certain degree, and is certainly up to bearing the loads and stresses of the normal flexion and extension of the knee over a long period of time. But in many people, particularly those with weak knee-extensor muscles in their thighs, it is not up to bearing the repeated stresses of jumping. Repeated jumping and improper landing will cause it to fatigue. When fatigue occurs, the tendon will be vulnerable to breakdown in the form of tears of its fibers. Inflammation of the tendon, and of the bone and muscles to which it is attached, follow. This is patellar tendinitis, or jumper's knee.

TREATMENT, CURE, AND PREVENTION
OF JUMPER'S KNEE

There are four simple ingredients in the treatment, cure, and prevention of jumper's knee. Although

severe cases may require surgery—similar to tennis-
elbow surgery—to relieve the constant stresses on the
patella and patellar tendon, most weekend-athlete
cases I have seen respond well to conservative therapy.

Fortunately, unlike ligaments, the tendons in our
body are capable of repairing themselves by generating
new tissue to replace torn fibers. Therefore, rest is the
first ingredient of treatment. Through rest, the torn
tendon will heal. That means abstaining from jumping
for awhile, and from any other abrupt knee extensions.

Once the tendon itself has healed, however, inflammation and pain may remain at its attachment to
the kneecap. If so, an appropriate dosage of cortisone
should solve the problem.

After the tendon has healed and all pain has subsided, your next job is to work toward preventing recurrence when you resume playing basketball or volleyball.* Remember, for everything pleasurable you
get in life, you must give something. Here the giving is,
again, a commitment to an exercise program designed
to strengthen your quadriceps muscles so that your
knees' tendency to hyperextend when jumping will be
lessened. Exercises 2 and 3 of the trick-knee exercises
I outlined on page 143 are the best home routines
you can do. I would not recommend Exercise 1, since
it puts too great an additional strain on your patellar
tendon.

Finally, you should learn to jump with just a shade
less gusto than you are used to. Even more importantly,
you *must* strive to land on your toes, that is, on the balls
of your feet, rather than flat-footed. At the same time,

---

*Patellar tendinitis can occur *in* other sports and can certainly interfere
with your enjoyment *of* other sports, such as skiing and tennis, but it is most
often seen in, and develops from, the jumping sports.

you should flex or bend your knees slightly in anticipation of landing so that some of the shocks and stresses of landing are absorbed by your knee's flexor muscles in the calf and thigh.

SURFER'S KNEE

Here is another painful ailment that involves the kneecap. The medical name for it is *prepatellar bursitis,* and in considering it we come to another component in the structure and function of the knee I haven't yet described. This component is the joint's lubricating system.

I have already said that the articulating surfaces of the bones of every joint in the body are covered by a coating of moist, membranous cartilage which reduces the friction between the surfaces and prevents wear and tear. In addition to these lubricative coatings, there are two other systems in and around the major joints whose functions are to provide further lubrication of the various parts. One is a series of *bursae* (plural of bursa); the other is the joint's *synovium.*

A *bursa* (from the Greek word for "pouch") is a flat membranous sac which overlies a bony prominence or tendon. Because its inner walls are moist, it prevents other structures around the tendon from rubbing directly against the tendon when it is in the act of moving a bone.

One of the principal bursae of the knee is the *prepatellar bursa.* The kneecap is a bone, but it is sheathed in tendinous tissue. More tendinous tissue passes over the kneecap as the quadriceps tendon blends into the top of the kneecap and emerges below as the patellar ligament, tying the kneecap to the tibia.

Every time the knee is flexed or extended, all these tissues move against one another. Therefore nature designed a bursa, or lubricating sac, to be inserted between the kneecap and the skin for the purpose of preventing rubbing of these parts. The bursa is located over, or in front of, the kneecap and thus is called the *prepatellar bursa.*

Under normal conditions, this bursa usually performs its lubricating function without any trouble. Again, it is only when abnormal stresses and loads are applied to it that difficulties arise. These difficulties occur in the form of inflammations of the bursa.

Abnormal stresses and loads do not come about through the movement of the quadriceps tendon or the kneecap, however. Rather, they come about through stresses the prepatellar bursa is really not designed to endure for any length of time. These are the stresses and pressures produced by extensive kneeling on hard surfaces or by sudden sharp blows directly on the bursa.

When we kneel, our knees are tightly flexed and the contact between them and the ground (or whatever else we are kneeling on) is made at the bottom of our kneecaps. In other words, the weight of our bodies is almost completely on the bottom of our kneecaps, causing them to push upward and their bursae to be excessively stressed. As a result, the bursae become inflamed and painful.

In the old days, the only extensive kneeling that was done was by religious worshipers and housemaids. Prayer benches were usually covered with cushion, but the floors on which housemaids toiled were bare and hard. Thus, the frequent cases of prepatellar bursitis that occurred came to be known as "housemaid's knee."

Today the only people who do any extensive kneeling on hard surfaces are surfers, so the ailment has come to be called "surfer's knee." I'm sure most of you have seen films of surfers kneeling on their surfboards for hours on end peering out to sea and waiting for the "big one." And I'm sure all of you who are surfers are more than familiar with the painful symptoms of prepatellar bursitis.

What causes surfer's knee? Well, we've seen that the *precipitating cause* is extensive kneeling on a hard surface, which produces excessive pressure on the bursa of the kneecap. The *underlying cause* is what comes after.

Extensive and unrelieved pressure on the prepatellar bursa causes it to become inflamed. The inner wall of the bursa is lined with cells that produce a thick, yellowish fluid that acts as a lubricant. Constant pressures irritate these cells. As they become inflamed they react by producing excess fluid. The excess fluid distends the normally flat bursa until it begins to look like a balloon filled with water.

If the knee is rested—that is, not knelt upon—the cellular inflammation subsides, further fluid is not secreted, and other cells will resorb the fluid, returning everything to normal. But if kneeling is continued— and surfer's are not famous for letting a bit of knee pain interfere with their pleasures—the condition will become chronic. The inflamed cells will produce further excess fluid, the bursa's distension will increase, and it will press against adjoining structures. The danger here is that tiny nodules will begin to grow on the surface of the bursa. These nodules cause the bursa to remain inflamed and swollen, and various knee motions will become agonizing. In addition, any pressure, however gentle, will produce pain.

The condition known as "surfer's knobs" is an outgrowth of surfer's knee. This is a condition in which it appears that large bubbles are encased within the skin just in front of the kneecaps. These bubbles are, of course, the chronically swollen and malfunctioning prepatellar bursae.

Surfer's knee is painful but, as many surfing enthusiasts will attest, endurable. If allowed to become chronic, however, it can create serious future knee problems. With almost constant pain over the tendinous and patellar areas in the front of the knee, the victim will tend to alter the way he moves his knee. Such alterations will put new stresses on other components of the joint, especially along the articulating surfaces, which can result in abnormal wear and tear and arthritis. So, it is the greater part of wisdom to avoid letting surfer's knee become chronic.

The best treatment is rest, after which one should employ knee pads—admittedly unglamorous, but vital —when returning to surfing. Cortisone can be used to reduce inflammation and hasten healing; in stubborn cases, when the swollen and blocked bursa refuses to resorb fluid, the fluid can be drained with a needle. Occasionally, the condition becomes so irritating, however, that the damaged bursa must be completely removed surgically. But that's OK because Mother Nature simply produces another healthy bursa to take its place.

WATER ON THE KNEE

Speaking of fluid brings us to our fourth major ailment of the knee—the condition popularly, and incorrectly, known as "water on the knee." It also brings us to that other important component of the knee joint: the *synovium*.

Completely encapsulating the knee joint—that is, its articulating surfaces—is a thin pouchlike membrane which secretes fluid into the joint, nourishes the articular cartilage, and further aids in its lubrication. This membrane is called the synovium. The synovium is overlaid with, and protected by, a layer of dense, tough, fibrous tissue; this overlay is called the capsule of the knee. The capsule not only protects the synovial membrane, it also acts as an additional brace and support for the knee. However, we are now concerned with the function of the synovium.

The synovium is fed by the body's blood-supply system. As blood passes through the synovial membrane it produces in the membrane's tissues a clear plasma dialysate which then seeps into the joint and is resorbed, constantly lubricating and nourishing the interior parts of the joint. As with the bursa of the kneecap, when the synovium becomes irritated, due to some abnormality or prolonged stress, the cells become inflamed and it swells, causing an excess of synovial fluid to fill the joint. And if the synovium is severely traumatized, blood will seep through its pores and join the fluid filling the joint.

This, in essence, is the condition known as water on the knee. Of course, the appellation is an inaccurate one: what occurs is not water on the knee but *excessive synovial fluid in* the knee.

Water on the knee in its chronic form usually comes about when a chronic abnormality in the knee causes the synovial membrane to swell and release excess amounts of synovial fluid into the knee joint itself.

The excess fluid creates a kind of hydraulic or outward-expanding pressure on the interior surfaces of the joint, which in itself produces further pain and may limit motion.

Treatment and relief are twofold in their objectives. First is the relief of the immediate condition by aspirating the knee, that is, draining the excess fluid by means of a needle. Second is the identification and treatment of the abnormality in the knee that has provoked the swelling of the synovial membrane and its discharge of fluid.

Water on the knee is really the *symptom* of an ailment rather than the ailment itself—except in rare cases. If your knee ever has the occasion to swell and feel distended and "heavy" without any apparent cause, you can be sure that there is an underlying disorder within your knee joint that you might not be aware of. It could be anything from an inflammation in some part of the knee to an infection, and you should have it examined by your physician immediately.

DANCER'S KNEE

Dancer's knee is known medically as *patellar chondromalacia,* which means a softening of the articular cartilage on the undersurface of the kneecap. It occurs most frequently among young women, especially those who take up ballet dancing as a form of exercise. The reason is most probably due to the fact that a woman's pelvic girdle is wider than a man's. Therefore, her thigh bones meet her knees at a more acute angle, forcing her knees inward and causing her to be slightly knock-kneed. This natural knock-kneed configuration causes an unequal pull on the kneecap when the knee is bent—one side of the kneecap, the inside, gets pulled higher than the outside by the quadriceps muscles each time the knee is bent and straightened. The condition also occurs in knock-kneed men as well.

You'll recall that the underside of the kneecap articulates with the front of the knee joint. To do this, it has a layer of articular cartilage—the hard, rubbery, glistening substance attached to the bone. As the kneecap is pulled unequally, its articulation becomes irregular, and the articular cartilage becomes inflamed. It reacts by softening, which produces further inflammation and deep knee-pain. A piece of the cartilage may even tear off and float free within the joint, causing locking and other instabilities.

Treatment consists of rest and an injection or two of cortisone to reduce the inflammation. Usually the condition will heal by itself, and the prevention of further episodes will be aided by quadriceps strengthening exercises 2 and 3, outlined on page 143. If it does not heal, then surgery is indicated. Surgery consists of scraping away the softened articular cartilage and allowing new cartilage to grow in its place. During surgery, we also relax the uneven tension on the kneecap so that future articulation will be more normal.

6

YOUR BACK MISERIES

"Oh, my aching back!" is one of the most commonly heard laments of weekend athletes. If recent figures from the National Center for Health Statistics—which reflect the fact that over seven million Americans are currently being treated by physicians for chronic back ailments—are correct, the chances are very good that you have a back problem. Why? Because the majority of people who develop garden-variety back ailments do so as a consequence of some strenuous physical activity, frequently in the field of sports.

Back ailments account for the third most frequent occurrence of sports-connected physical miseries in this country. And with sports participation soaring at the rate it is, the rate of back-pain complaints is rising proportionately. It is my guess that within five years, back afflictions will lead the parade. This is sad to observe, because in many ways back problems, of all sports-related disorders, are the easiest to prevent. All it takes, really, is an increased awareness on the part of weekend athletes of how their backs operate and how to prepare their backs for the athletic movements and maneuvers to which they are unaccustomed.*

As a practicing orthopedic surgeon with years of experience in dealing with back problems, I can assure the great majority of you that you need not endure the pain, misery, and frequent disability you are forced to suffer as a result of your faulty backs. Most of your problems are due in the first place to ignorance and mismanagement. The great majority of back ailments I am required to treat, whether surgically or by more conservative means, could have been avoided in the very beginning through the application of a little practical knowledge and common sense when the first ache or spasm appeared.

Unfortunately, the very people who will rush their Cadillacs and Lincolns off to the mechanic at the first sign of a rattling shock absorber or squeaking spring will not be as faithful to themselves after their first episode of back pain. Yet their backs are more valuable to them than a lifetime's worth of fine and expensive cars.

But enough preaching. Later in this chapter I will tell you what you need to do to help ensure the prevention of common sports-derived back miseries. Let me now turn to the miseries themselves.

---

*Everything you need to know about your back, its pain and its relief, can be found in my book *Oh, My Aching Back!*, published in 1973 by David McKay Co., Inc., New York. In this chapter I will only discuss the miseries that commonly derive from sports.

GETTING TO KNOW YOUR BACK

Your back constitutes the largest single part of your body and contains the most moving parts. It follows, then, that your back is subject to more malfunctions than any other region of your anatomy.

Basically, the human back is a framework capable of either great flexibility or stubborn rigidity, depending on the dictate of circumstances. From this framework every other part of the body is suspended or otherwise supported. Every part of the body relates to the back in one way or another.

The principal structure of the back, the spine, is just about the first piece of operating machinery an embryo grows as it blossoms within its mother's womb. The spine's awesomely complex, but perfectly organized, system of neurological networks directly controls every function of the body from the neck down, and more than a few from the neck up as well. Its precisely formed bones—called *vertebrae*—are sturdily linked, one to the other, by some of the strongest and most durable ligaments to be found in the body.

Within and surrounding the spine, and enabling it to function in the many ways it does, is a vast network of nerves, blood vessels, bones, ligaments, cartilage, tendons, and muscles. Except for direct injuries to, or defects in, the spine itself, most back ailments develop as a result of weaknesses in the spine-associated structures, *especially in the muscles* that support and move it.

Let's have a closer look at your spine and see what its architecture is all about and what makes it so unique and important in your life. First of all, keep in mind that it serves three main purposes:

1. It is the support structure for your body, an-
    choring your ribs and connecting your head
    with your pelvis and legs.
2. It is the housing for your spinal cord, which is
    the link between your brain and the rest of
    your body.
3. It is the primary instrument of your body's
    flexibility.

For purposes of illustration, we can divide the
spine into four regions. These regions are identified by
the specific characteristics of their vertebrae. We find,
then:

1. *The Cervical Spine, or Neck Region.* This area
    consists of seven vertebrae. The main charac-
    teristics of the cervical vertebrae are their ex-
    traordinary range of motion. In addition to
    supporting the head, their mobility permits
    the head and neck to rotate through a wide
    spectrum. The base of the skull is connected
    by ligaments to the top of the cervical spine,
    and by tendons to many of the motor muscles
    of the neck and upper shoulder. Situated be-
    tween each of the seven cervical vertebrae,
    and conforming to their shapes, are "discs"—
    gel-filled, cartilage-walled capsules which act
    as cushions between the vertebrae and aid in
    the articulation of each *intervertebral joint.**
2. *The Thoracic or Dorsal Spine, or Mid-Back Re-
    gion.* Twelve vertebrae, called the thoracic

---

*The spaces between each of the twenty-six vertebrae of the entire spine
constitute joints, insofar as each of the vertebrae articulate with their immediate neighbors. Thus, the spine is a series of joints which have the same
components—muscles, ligaments, tendons, etc.—as the other joints of the
body.

vertebrae, form this region. They are similar in shape and function to the cervical verte- brae, but are progressively larger. They are also separated and cushioned by discs which conform to their shape. Special connections are present for the attachment of the twelve ribs. Because of the rib-attaching function, this area of the spine is relatively immobile.

3. *The Lumbar Spine, or Lower-Back Region.* The brunt of the weight of the upper body is borne by the five large vertebrae, the *lumbar vertebrae,* in this region. They are broader and heavier than the ones above in order to sup- port the weight and mass of the torso. In addi- tion, very large muscles associated with the back, abdomen, and hips attach to these verte- brae. They too are separated by discs, and it is in this part of the spine that most back ail- ments are centered.

4. *The Sacrum and Coccyx Region.* The *sacrum* constitutes the base of the spine. It is a broad, triangular bone attached at its top to the lum- bar spine and on its sides to the pelvis. In the development of the spine in the embryo, the sacrum consists of five separate bones. They eventually fuse together into the single sac- rum. The *coccyx* (pronounced "cox-ix") is the collection of a few small bones which protrude from the lower end of the sacrum. These bones are probably the remnants of what was once man's tail in his early evolutionary period. The coccyx is the site of a misery familiar to all ice skaters and certain other sports enthusiasts.

The spine is not all there is to the bone structure of the back. On each of its two sides the sacrum attaches to two large fan-shaped bones called *ilia*. The *ilia* curve around toward the front of the body and connect to each other in front to form the pelvis—the spine's foundation and its go-between to the legs.

As you see, the spine is made of bones. But man is more than bones. If we view the spine as being similar to the foundation of a house, we know that the blocks of the foundation must be cemented together to be an effective supporting base. In the case of your spine, the mortar that holds the dry foundation bricks, the bones, together is your ligaments, cartilages, tendons, and muscles. When put together, the entire package amounts to a mechanism that can bend and twist, turn and squirm, shake and wriggle, and do just about anything else within the range of human motion—as long as it remains healthy. Just as easily, it can stiffen up, hold itself rigid in a variety of positions, or exert peak power whenever required—again, as long as it remains healthy.

Numerous ligaments connect and hold the foundation blocks of the spine together. A few of these deserve a closer look because of the disability and pain they can produce if they are damaged by excessive motion in the back.

1.   *The Interspinous Ligaments.* The *interspinous ligaments* are bands of tough ligamentous tissue that hold each of the vertebrae together along their *spinous processes*. (The spinous processes of the vertebrae are the protrusions you can feel just under your skin when you run your fingers up and down your spine.) These ligaments relax when we *extend* our spines (bend backward) but become tight when we

flex them (bend forward), and thus help to limit the motion that can occur between each of the vertebrae. Occasionally, when sudden severe flexion of the spine occurs—and it usually occurs in the neck region—one or more of these ligaments may tear, or rupture, and cause localized pain and misery for long periods of time.

2. *The Anterior and Posterior Longitudinal Ligaments.* The *anterior* and *posterior longitudinal ligaments* run the length of the spine, one in front of the bodies of the vertebrae and one behind. The "bodies" are the round, flat bones that constitute the main portion of each vertebra. Between each body is situated a disc. The bodies constitute the front part of the spine. Branching rearward from each vertebral body are three bony spurs which are the articulating surfaces of the intervertebral joints. Two spurs branch laterally and are called the *transverse processes,* one spur branches rearward and is called the *spinous process,* which I have already mentioned as being that portion of your spine you can feel with your fingers. Separating the main body of each vertebra from its articulating spurs is a hole called the *vertebral foramen.* With the twenty-six vertebrae stacked one on top of another, these holes run as one long tunnel through the core of the spine. Through it travels the spinal cord. The arch that surrounds the foramen and connects the vertebral spurs to the main body of each vertebra is called the *lamina.*

So, then, the *anterior longitudinal ligament* runs the length of the spine *in front of* the vertebral bodies, connecting them along the way anteriorly. And the *posterior longitudinal ligament* runs the length of the spine *behind* the vertebral bodies, but in front of the spinal cord as it travels through the vertebral foramen. The posterior ligament connects the bodies of the vertebrae posteriorly, or behind, and both the anterior and posterior ligaments help hold the intervertebral discs in place. These are not the only things these two ligaments do, but for our purposes here we need not concern ourselves with their other functions.

Of all the ligaments along the spine, the anterior longitudinal ligament is most susceptible to tearing in sudden extension overloads. Such injuries occur most frequently in the neck during "whiplash" stresses. These episodes take place most frequently in everyday life during automobile accidents, when one car is struck from behind and its occupants' heads are abruptly jerked backward. The new, high-backed seats of late model cars have partly solved this problem in many accidents, but it still occurs.

Whiplash can and often does occur in various sports activities as well, particularly sports in which there is a good deal of physical contact. The most familiar of these comes about in football when one player "clothes-lines" an opponent, that is, swings his stiffened arm across the front of the opponent's helmet. However, sudden involuntary whiplash stresses can happen in less violent athletic activities, too—in tennis, for instance, when jerking the neck back to make an overhead smash, or in springboard diving when faulty impact is made with the water. A little knowledge about your spinal ligaments and how much they can endure should be of some help in avoiding these neck-region injuries and the long-term miseries that flow from them.

The posterior longitudinal ligament—the one that travels along the rear portions of the vertebral bodies and intervertebral discs—presents its own problems. I will get to these in a few moments.

There are many more ligaments in and around the spine, and they are all subject to injury and chronic pain. However, our subject is not so much injuries to the spine as it is sports-connected ailments of the back, so I shall move along to the primary villain in back miseries—the muscles. As you will learn, the muscles of the back (notice that I didn't say the muscles *in* the back) bear much of the blame for sports-derived back miseries. And these same muscles, if strengthened and conditioned, can prevent a great percentage of back pain and Monday-morning remorse.

If you wanted to hold a long pole vertically erect with three guy wires, each wire would have to exert a pull equal to each of the other two. But if one wire is weak, or slack, regardless of how strong the other two are the pole will not remain vertical. It will sag in the direction of the other two wires—an abnormal motion.

Your spine acts similarly. There are three basic muscle groups that not only move your spine but also support it, and help to hold it erect. These are like the wires in my pole analogy. When one muscle group grows weak through disuse, abnormal motion of the spine occurs, the other two groups are forced to do most of the work, and fatigue, strain, and pain follow. Moreover, damage to the spine itself is likely.

The three basic muscle groups which support the spine are:

1. *The Extensor Muscles*
2. *The Lateral Muscles*
3. *The Abdominal Muscles*

Are you surprised that I include the abdominal muscles? Many people are when I mention it. They shouldn't be, however, since it only makes sense that the back must have some support in front of it.

The abdominal muscles support your abdominal wall. They extend from your rib cage to the sides and front of your pelvis. They consist of several different muscle groups, each with its own primary function, but since they all interact, we can consider them as a unit. These muscles, in addition to supporting the contents of your abdominal cavity, help to control the bending, or flexing, movements of your spine—every time you bend forward your spine is pulled by your abdominals. And when they are tensed, they help to relieve strains on your back, as when you lift something. Let's consider them as your anterior guy wires.

The extensor muscles lie along the spine itself and are also known as the *spine extensors,* which means they are mainly responsible for your ability to extend your back, or bend backward. They consist of many layers of muscle with complicated names which we need not go into here. Some of the muscles, however, are very small and span short distances, in certain cases only an inch. Others are vast and extend from your

neck to your sacrum. Generally, the larger spine extensors lie close to your skin, while the smaller ones are
nearer the bones. But they all act in concert to move
and support your back. They get their heaviest play
when you arch your back, hold your spine stiff and erect
as when standing at attention, or push or pull some
heavy weight.

The lateral, or side, muscles are pretty well hidden.
They lie against the lateral aspects of your spine and
control the side-bending of your back. One of them, the
psoas major muscle, is one of the largest single muscles
in your body. It is present on both sides of your spine;
it passes from the spine through the pelvis and attaches
to the top inner part of the thigh bone just below the
hip joint. Thus it affects not only your back but plays a
role in the movements of your hips and legs as well. It
is called a "two-joint" muscle because it acts on more
than one joint. It is also one of the chief villains in back
pain, since it is the muscle most frequently subject to
overloads and strains.

Although the abdominals, spine extensors, and
spine laterals are the three major muscle groups involved in the movement and support of your back,
there is a fourth group that plays an important role too
—despite the fact that it is not located in the back. This
group is composed of a collection of muscles in your
hips.

Another surprise? It shouldn't be, when you think
about it. By virtue of the close relationship of your hips
to your pelvis, and that of your pelvis to your spine,
what goes on in your hips can have a very significant
effect on your back. First of all, we have already seen
that your *psoas major* muscle travels from the side of
your back through your hips. But the principal hip mus-

cles themselves—those which move your hip joints—
also involve your back because every time you move
your hips, stresses are placed on your back muscles and
spine.

The four principal muscle groups in your hips are
the *hip flexors*, the *hip abductors* (those which enable
you to spread your legs), the *hip adductors* (those
which enable you to close your legs), and the *hip extensors*. Each of the four groups consists of several different individual muscles; all work together in the movement of your hips, and all have an effect on your back.
However, the group that involves your back most significantly is the *hip extensors*.

Your hip extensors are the massive muscles that lie
along the back of your hip joint. The most prominent
muscle in this group is the *gluteus maximus*. It exists as
a pair, known among bodybuilders and weight lifters as
"the glutes." They form the major portion of your der-
riere and are the muscles you contract when you
tighten your buttocks. As they pass behind your hip
they become the main muscles you use when you climb
stairs. Running power and speed come from this muscle
too.

The hip extensors as a group control *lumbar lordosis*, the natural curve of your lumbar spine, which,
when excessive, produces "swayback," a condition
painfully present in many people. These muscles, when
combined with the *hip flexors*, are extremely important in maintaining good posture.

Poor posture is without a doubt the principal *underlying cause* of most common back ailments. Poor
posture places a chronic, weakening strain on the muscles of the back, reducing their ability to support the
spine. Thus, when a *precipitating cause* is present, such

as a severe twisting or wrenching injury, not only are the back muscles subject to damage, but the ligaments and bones of the spine as well. You can see, then, that your hip muscles are vital to a healthy back.

Taken together—your backbone, the ligaments that hold it all together, and the muscles, tendons, and bones that support it—your back is quite a remarkable hunk of machinery; it is as delicate as a fine Swiss watch and as tough as a Mack truck. Given proper care, a fair shake, and a little understanding, your back will take on any job you ask of it, including most of the fantastic contortions it is put through in many sports.

When it fails, the failure in practically all of the most severe cases arises out of some weakness in one or more of its various components—again, the *underlying-cause* factor. Such an unhappy condition is generally called "back instability," and when instability occurs, the odds are good that it will launch a virulent case of *lumbago, sciatica,* or some other form of back misery. And when worse comes to worst, there will be the nastiest of all afflictions to deal with: "slipped disc."

SLIPPED DISC

As I've indicated, back ailments tend to be progressive; that is, except in cases of severe and sudden injury, most chronic sports-associated back disorders evolve from the combination of weak outer back muscles and strains to those muscles, and then go on to develop into recurring, deeper muscle strains as the larger supporting muscles lose their ability to support the spine fully.

The progressive weakening of the back eventually works its way down to the spine itself, so that the vertebrae of the spinal column—especially in the most-weight-bearing lumbar region—undergo slight but significant changes in their relationships to each other. This in turn places unaccustomed strains on their ligaments. As the ligaments weaken the vertebrae and all their parts experience further relational distortions. Once this condition is reached, it takes only a minor twist or strain to unleash a whole new kind of havoc—the slipped disc.

A "slipped disc" neither slips, nor is it a disc, but because we are all accustomed to the phrase by now I'll continue to use it. The affliction popularly known as slipped disc is in reality a complete breakdown of an *intervertebral joint* in the spine, for that is what a disc is. Slipped disc can and often does occur in the neck, or cervical region, of the spine, but its most frequent site is in the lumbar spine. This, again, is because this portion of the spine bears most of your upper-body weight.

Although not the most common cause of back pain, faulty discs are by far the biggest source of serious back trouble from a percentage standpoint. Along with those cases definitely identifiable during diagnosis as disc problems, there are many back disorders that are traceable to the discs but are not sufficiently advanced to show up as such. That is why it is so important that you start looking after your back once you've had your first episode of pain. Most severe disc problems—the ones that end up on the operating table—get that way because they are neglected in their early stages. The best way to head off the development of a mild back problem into a severe and agonizing disc disorder is, of course, through exercise, by strengthening the muscles of your back and taking some of the load off your spinal column.

I will detail a few exercises that are effective in achieving this objective a few pages ahead, but to appreciate their value you should first know something about your discs and what exactly happens when they "slip."

An intervertebral disc is a circular capsule which fills the space between each of the bodies of the vertebrae in your spine. It is composed of three distinct elements:

1. The top and bottom surfaces of each disc consist of plates of gristlelike cartilage which conform to the shape of the bodies of the two vertebrae to which the disc is joined. The joining of the discs to the vertebrae comes about through the blending of their fibers with the fibers of the vertebral bodies.

2. The second element consists of tough, elastic, ligamentous bands which, attached to the top and bottom plates, form the rounded wall of the capsule. These bands are overlaid in strips —obliquely and radially to one another like the plys of an automobile tire—to an average thickness of about one-eighth of an inch. (The rear portions of the wall are thinner than the front portions, and therein lies much of the source of disc troubles.) This wall is called the *annulus fibrosus,* and its elasticity allows the capsule to alter its shape in response to forces placed on it, then return to its normal shape.

3. Inside the capsule is the third element of the disc—the *nucleus pulposis,* which means "pulpy core." The pulpy core is a white, glistening, gel-like substance. This substance moves around within the confines of the cap-

sule's wall and acts hydraulically to provide the elastic capsule with a cushioning or shock-absorbing capability.

Although most laymen tend to think of the disc as being the entire capsule, medically speaking only the pulpy core is the disc. When you hear of a disc being removed by surgery, it is only the core that is removed, not the capsule itself. And when you hear of a "slipped disc," what is meant is that at least a portion of the pulpy core has somehow escaped from the capsule, not that the capsule itself has become displaced. Which brings us to the question of precisely what occurs when a disc slips.

The disc and its capsule have several functions in the spinal column, but the shock-absorbing one is the first among equals. With each movement of the spine, the disc-capsules expand and compress in various directions, depending on the direction of the motion, in order to reduce and absorb the shock waves that radiate through the spine with such movements.

Bending forward, or flexion, for instance, will cause the front portions of the lumbar discs to compress and the rear portions to widen—because flexion in the spine compresses the fronts of the vertebral bodies. All other motions create corresponding changes in the capsules' configuration. The capsules are able to act as shock absorbers, then, because their pulpy cores—the discs themselves—are compressible. Although the discs will adopt any odd shape in response to an outside force, i.e., flexion or extension in any direction, they cannot be expelled from their containers, the ligamentous capsules. Under normal conditions, that is.

But when abnormal conditions are present, one or

two discs *can* be expelled from their capsules. When this happens, we have what is known as slipped disc.

There are basically two abnormal conditions that lead to slipped disc. The first is a sudden, severe, traumatic injury, such as usually occurs in a fall from a high place or in an automobile accident. The second is a progressive weakening along the surface of the wall of the disc's capsule brought about by a constant strain on the spine, and it is this which we are concerned with here.

Remember, I said earlier that the wall of the capsule, the *annulus fibrosus,* tends to be thinner along its posterior aspect—the surface that faces the spinal cord as it travels down the spine between the bodies and the articulating spurs of the vertebrae—than along its anterior aspect. Add to that the fact that, as we age, the fluids in our body tend to dry up. But our discs' cores are essentially fluid. Hence, as we grow older the cores lose their gel-like quality and harden. The combination of inherently thinner rear capsule walls and progressively hardening pulpy cores sets the stage for slipped disc. When excessive lumbar lordosis is introduced into this recipe of nature, the stage is not only set, but the curtain begins to rise.

Lumbar lordosis, as I have said, is the natural inward curve of the lumbar spine. The adult spine has four curves: the *cervical curve* of the neck, which is a back-to-front curve; the *dorsal curve,* which continues the cervical curve but reverses it into a front-to-back curve; the *lumbar curve,* which carries the spine back into an inward-curving direction at the small of the back just above the buttocks region; and the *sacral curve,* which completes the spine outwardly again at its tip.

When looked at from the side, the spinal column looks like a "lazy-S," with the dorsal and lumbar curves the equivalents of the two major curves of the "S." In the dorsal region, the vertebrae and their discs are relatively immobile because of their attachments to the ribs. The vertebrae and discs in the cervical and lumbar regions are exposed to the most motion, and therefore to the most compression. But because the lumbar region supports much more weight, its discs receive even more compression than those in the neck.

Again, under normal circumstances the lumbar discs are easily capable of performing their hydraulic or shock-absorbing function. But when a permanent excessive lumbar lordosis exists—that is, when the lumbar curve is exaggerated—the compression of the front portions of the lumbar discs becomes abnormal.

Unless there is a genetic or organic defect in the spine, the lumbar curve usually becomes exaggerated because the back's supporting muscles have grown too weak to hold the curve in its normal shape. There is an increasingly permanent compression of the front portions of the lumbar discs as the bodies of the vertebrae pinch together, and a corresponding widening of the rear portions of the discs.

The gel-like discs, perhaps already beginning to dry out and harden through age (slipped discs increase in incidence with age up to fifty), are pressed against the rear walls of their capsules. Because the rear, or posterior, sector of the walls are naturally thinner than the front portions of the capsules, and because they are stretched as a result of the compression in front, they are required to endure greater tension than normal. Couple this with the pressure of the hardening discs within being forced against them, and you have the makings of one or more slipped discs.

What happens when a disc slips? It is really very simple. The core, pressing against the stretched and weakened posterior wall of the capsule, eventually causes fibers in the wall to tear. The wall of the capsule thereby loses its ability to contain the core. If the fibers of the wall are only partially torn, the core, or disc, will create a bulge at some point along the rear surface of the wall. This is called a *protruded disc.* The protrusion will grow with further compression of the front portion of the disc and will eventually bulge through the posterior longitudinal ligament, which, you'll remember, travels the length of the spine, holds the rear portions of the vertebral bodies together, and separates them from the spinal cord itself. Once the protrusion bulges through this ligament, it will press on the spinal cord, or on nerve roots branching out from it.

If the fibers of the capsule wall are completely torn, the core, or disc, will actually pop out of the capsule. This is called a *ruptured,* or *extruded, disc.* With its pulpy core extruded through the capsule, the intervertebral space will collapse, placing new strains on the spinal column. What is worse, the extruded material will then press on the spinal cord or on nerve roots branching out from it.

Most protruded discs do not occur directly in the rear of the capsule wall, but rather on one side or the other of the rear midline. Thus, the protrusion or extrusion usually encroaches upon the spinal canal on one side or the other. The result is that only the nerves on one side are compressed; hence pain and disability occur only on one side of the body. On those rarer occasions when the protrusion is directly rearward, pain can attack both sides at once.

As I have said, the most common site of a slipped disc is in the lumbar spine, especially in the discs of the two or three lowermost vertebrae. This is also the area in which the nerve roots which form the sciatic nerve emerge from the spinal cord and branch down through each leg to innervate the muscles of the lower extremities. Thus the terms *sciatica* and *lumbago,* which many people believe are ailments in themselves but which are actually only symptoms of a slipped disc.

Sciatica is severe pain in the lower back or buttocks region which radiates down one or both legs and into the feet due to irritation of the sciatic nerve. Such pain is usually a clear symptom of a disc disorder.

Lumbago, its twin, is severe pain in the lower back often accompanied by "locking" sensations, the feeling that the back has "gone out," and acute muscle spasm. It is caused by irritation of the sensory nerves in the region which, as in our earlier hot-stove illustration, send messages to the brain requesting relief. The brain activates the motor nerves; but because there is no finger to be lifted, the motor nerves cause the muscles they supply to go into states of uncontrolled contraction, or spasm. Lumbago is sometimes a symptom of slipped disc, but not always. It can also point to arthritis in the spine, or simply to strained muscles from poor spinal curvature or from unaccustomed activity.

When the ailment is slipped disc, the uncontrollable spasms of the lower-back muscles are extremely painful, but they are nature's way of helping the disorder to heal because they limit the movement of the spine and prevent more of the disc's pulpy core from being displaced. If further displacement is stopped, a kind of semi-healing will spontaneously take place by virtue of a scarring-over of the protrusion. The scarring will tend to hold the bulge in place, but only against normal pressures. If further excessive stresses are placed on the spine, as they usually are, then the bulge will expand. Once the disc protrudes it cannot go back into its capsule. It can only protrude more when the capsule is further squeezed. So it pays the person with signs of an even moderately slipped disc to treat his back with great care. The alternative, sooner or later, is the operating table.

This doesn't mean that the victim should become inactive, however. After years of recurrent disc-associated pain, a new kind of back problem may emerge. This is the pain which occurs with inactivity—the kind in which the sufferer finds that his or her back stiffens up unless it is kept supple and warm with constant motion. It is characteristic of this kind of pain that it is always worse after the back has been at rest, and mornings are usually the worst time for it. This pain is a symptom of spinal arthritis, which often develops out of long-term, recurrent disc trouble. It develops because the back muscles are allowed to grow lax, which creates uneven and intensified wear and tear on the intervertebral joints of the spine.

THE TREATMENT OF SLIPPED DISC

Setting aside for the moment slipped discs caused by direct accidents, we've seen that the condition is commonly a progressive one. It appears first as a mild, aching discomfort in the lower back. At this point, most sufferers tend to ignore it—thinking of it as just another twinge and perhaps settling for a bit of liniment and an easy chair.

Let's say you are the person I'm describing. There may even be the realization that the little wrench you gave your back yesterday when you were trying to blast out of some thick rough, or when you lost your balance getting off the ski lift, had something to do with your mild pain. What has actually happened inside your back, though, may have been the beginning of the end. A few small fibers in the wall of one of your discs might have been stretched or pulled beyond their capacity, perhaps aided by the progressive weakening of tissue that has been building up over the years as a result of your sloppy posture and flaccid back-support muscles.

A few days or maybe a week later, let's say, you're putting out the trash or lifting a bundle of wet laundry. This time the pain comes a little quicker and stronger —you have stretched a few more fibers in the faulty disc wall.

Things can go along like this for months, even years, getting progressively worse and lasting a little longer each time, until one day—Pow! Something happens that really knocks your back for a loop. That something can be as simple and commonplace as a sneeze or a cough. Or it can be leaning into your car to pull out your golf bag. Or reaching up to hit a tennis serve. This time neither liniment nor an easy chair helps. Your back is gripped by agonizing spasms. The pain you experience is giant sized. It is not economy sized, though, because now it's going to cost you time and money.

Starting with those few weak and stretched capsule fibers that started to break down way-back-when, one of your discs has collapsed, perhaps even ruptured. The pulpy core may already have started to squeeze through the rupture. If so, everybody is in for a hard time.

Especially you!

As the star of this unhappy and painful drama, you,

the patient, will find yourself in bed, usually lying on one side with your legs pulled up to your chest to relieve the pressure on the afflicted nerve. The tired, weary muscles of your back, constantly straining to find some position of comfort, will begin to ache of their own account from the effort.

If the damage to your disc is the result of an accident of some kind, there is at least one small advantage —you'll probably get immediate attention and treatment, without waiting, without trying to kid yourself that it's really not all that serious. You will thereby be launched on the long job of getting well that much sooner.

No matter what the cause, once the diagnosis has been made that one of your discs has begun to protrude, the first phase of treatment must be complete bed rest in order to relieve all strain on the area and give the disc a chance to stabilize and heal. If you were to continue to stand on your feet, the weight of your body would compress the affected disc and cause additional protrusion. This would sooner or later lead to complete rupture of the capsule if it hadn't already happened.

By complete bed rest I mean *complete bed rest.* That means no sitting up to take meals, no getting up to use the bathroom or to take a shower because you can't stand yourself another moment. If this is impossible to achieve at home, then you should undergo it in a hospital. It's true that some patients with disc damage manage to break the rules without serious consequences. However, you don't want to take chances with your back, and the most you have to lose is a little time in exchange for giving the damaged disc a chance to heal.

If you were my patient I would definitely suggest hospitalization in any case of disc protrusion. Since lying on your back with your legs straight out is not the best form of rest-treatment for protruded discs, I would arrange to use a routine pelvic traction device. If you've heard about traction you are likely to have an image of some torturous medieval device which stretches your spine and causes all sorts of additional agonies. Your fears would be unfounded. The type of traction I would employ is a simple device consisting of a girdlelike belt which wraps around your waist and hips. Straps are attached to the sides and each strap is in turn attached to weights which hang over the foot of the bed. I use approximately ten pounds of weight for each strap, lowering or raising the amount of weight depending on the size of the patient.

Traction is not intended to stretch or pull your vertebrae apart in order to allow the disc to "slip" back into place, as many people suppose. The disc *will not slip back*. The purpose of the traction is to raise your pelvis and reduce the curve in your lumbar spine, thereby relieving the pressure of the protruded disc on your nerves and relieving muscle spasm. Sorry to deflate the myth about traction—it is only an aid to treatment, not treatment itself.

Along with traction, I would give you pain medication and muscle relaxants. Hot packs applied to the affected region are sometimes helpful, but their use is really limited. X rays and blood tests would be done, and I would be able to examine you daily and evaluate your progress. If no evidence of nerve-root damage existed, I would then concern myself with reducing your muscle spasm. If there were neurological changes, these would have to be watched very carefully.

After about ten or twelve days of this type of bed rest, with good progress on your part—absence of spasms, return of sensation and motor power, and obvious improvement in your general comfort—I would then start to gradually put you on your feet. Initially, you would be allowed out of bed twice a day for ten minutes. If you tolerated this well, I would slowly increase the duration of standing and walking. But I would permit no immediate sitting down, except for the bathroom.

You would simultaneously begin gentle exercises in bed. Over the next seven or eight days you should progress to the point where you can be up for an hour or so without discomfort—the minimum requirement for discharge and going home. In order to function at home, even on a minimal level, you must be able to tolerate being out of bed for at least one hour. Sitting is always the most strenuous activity for your back except for bending and lifting, so I would have you delay doing any sitting for a long time.

Once home, you would continue daily to increase your activities and add specific exercises to your regimen. When you are able to be up and about most of the day (this takes two to three weeks), you could consider returning to work on a part-time basis if your work was not strenuous and if it did not require much traveling.

It now becomes clear that a real slipped disc, treated without an operation, requires about six to eight weeks in order to heal sufficiently to enable you to return to even part-time normal activities.

Is that a big sigh I hear? Well, the best treatment is to prevent the entire problem in the first place, which only you can do. I have described the general conservative postdiagnosis treatment. Of course, there are exceptions. Some people are better in one week, while others may require six weeks of bed rest and traction. Notice, I have not prescribed a single back brace.

What happens if you don't get better? The spasms continue, the neurological changes persist or even get worse—what then? Since I have been seeing you every day, I am well aware that you are not improving. At the end of a week with no improvement, I would obtain a myelogram.* (In the presence of serious neurological deficits, I would have had a myelogram done immediately when you were admitted.) If the myelogram confirms the presence of large disc protrusion, I would then feel it necessary to proceed with surgery and remove the disc. But if the myelogram does not reveal a herniation of the disc or if it shows that the defect is very slight, I would continue with bed rest and traction for an additional period of time.

Each disc patient I treat has his or her own particular physiological nature, and everyone's degree of disc damage differs from everyone else's. This makes it very difficult to predict the outcome of a disc problem, but I can say in general that of every hundred disc patients I see in my office, thirty of them will require hospitalization. Of these thirty patients, fifteen will need an operation. Before I describe disc operations and their results, two examples of the difficulty of diagnosis and prediction might be illuminating.

A middle-aged man, dynamic, successful, chairman of the board of a billion-dollar-a-year company, was brought to my office in excruciating pain. He was

---

*A myelogram is an X ray of your spine done with a dye injected painlessly into your spinal canal. It pinpoints the exact site of disc protrusion.

tilted to one side and his back spasms were so severe he could hardly talk. He was in too much pain for a thorough examination, but I was able to determine that his neurological system was intact. I had him immediately admitted to the hospital and placed on bed rest with pelvic traction. He was given adequate pain relievers and muscle relaxants. His X rays were normal. After three days, he was out of bed and walking. He had no pain, and returned to work the next day.

Remarkable? Yes, but he had severe lumbo-sacral spasm, probably associated with tension fatigue, poor posture, and excessive sitting. His attack had occurred while he was at a board meeting. His pencil had dropped to the floor and he leaned over sideways to pick it up. He felt a sudden contraction in his back and was unable to move. When giving his history, he told me that the pain was radiating into his leg, but upon further questioning I learned that the pain went down his thigh only to his knee, not below. Classical sciatic pain radiates all the way down the leg to the foot. Depending upon the nerve root involved, the pain may localize near the heel or near the big toe. So, then, this gentleman did not have a genuine disc protrusion and he recovered in a short time. However, I started him on an exercise program because he now had a definite lumbo-sacral weakness. The next time he strains his lower back, his disc may not hold up and might actually extrude, that is, slip. So a preventive program is necessary to strengthen his back and reduce the possibility of another strain.

Another patient, a forty-two-year-old, overweight female who was employed as a legal secretary, had been having bouts of back pain with radiation down her right leg to the foot for several years. She had been hospitalized twice, each time for three weeks. She had worn different types of braces almost continuously. She had had diathermy, injections, hot packs, even chiropractic manipulation. She told me that she had recently been seen by another orthopedist who had recommended surgery. She was absolutely terrified of surgery and would go to any length in order to avoid it.

Well, my examination revealed that she had moderate muscle spasm of her back, some atrophy of her right leg muscles with concurrent weakness, loss of ankle reflexes, and decreased sensation in her foot. I told her that in view of her history and symptoms she probably would require surgery, but that it would be worthwhile to try first extensive bed rest and traction. We tried for six weeks. At the end of the third week she was no better. She still had pain, and her neurological findings were unchanged.

A myelogram revealed a large bulging disc between the lowest lumbar vertebra and the sacrum. She still refused surgery. At the end of six weeks of complete bed rest without even bathroom privileges, she showed improvement. Her pain was almost gone. Her leg movements and other signs were improved, and her muscle tone was better. But sensation was still decreased. In another three weeks she was at home, on her exercise program. Eight weeks after her discharge she was back to work part-time, and at the end of sixteen weeks she was working full-time.

Now, she has not been cured. She still gets occasional back and leg pain and must rest at home for a few days. The numbness in her foot persists, and she continues to have a limp. Nevertheless, she is happy. She did not want an operation. She can work, and she tolerates her limitations in rather good spirits.

The moral of this story is that we treat the patient, not necessarily the disc. Contrary to much popular belief, most surgeons do not sit in their offices with scalpels in hand just waiting for disc cases to show up. We would much rather save a disc than excise it, if it is at all possible and practical. Whether we can or not often depends on the patient—whether he or she is willing to go through the long, quiescent period of treatment in bed.

SURGICAL TREATMENT

The decision of whether or not to operate is not difficult. In some instances the patient is so fed up with his pain, weakness, and disability that he practically begs for surgery. At other times the doctor must make the suggestion and explain the reasons for it. No one particularly enjoys undergoing surgery, yet there are times when this is the only sensible treatment.

Surgery would be called for in your case if you were to have persistent pain and it was not relieved by traction and bed rest, or if you were to have pronounced weakness and numbness of the leg, and the neurological deterioration was progressive.

What does the surgeon do? I'll spare you the gory details, but in essence he locates the disc herniation, either visually or by feel. He removes the extruded portion of the damaged disc, and then, with special instruments, extracts the remainder of the disc's pulp from the collapsed capsule.

"My goodness," patients often exclaim, "what happens to the empty space?" Not very much happens to the space. It is already very thin due to the collapse of the disc. After the disc is removed, the space gradually fills in with scar tissue. Obviously the scar tissue does not replace the function of the nucleus pulposis—it is not an efficient shock absorber—but it *will* fill up the space. Over a long period of time the space between the two vertebrae may also be bridged by bone tissue which grows between the vertebrae, creating a kind of spontaneous fusion which adds stability to the area.

I would emphasize here that treatment does not end with the removal of the damaged disc. Slipped disc, although a genuine disorder in itself, is also a symptom of a more insidious disorder—instability and weakness of the back in general. Removing the disc does not strengthen the back and erase its general instability. To achieve that takes, first, the healing process, and then a gradual building up of the back's supports once the patient has recovered from the effects of the surgery.

The success of a disc operation is dependent upon three things: competent surgery, good postoperative care, and faithful postoperative back therapy. The surgeon is responsible for carrying out the third part. Although I have never officially tabulated the results of my slipped disc operations, I would estimate that 85 percent of the patients I have operated on for this condition were able to resume their normal physical activities (I exclude strenuous sports like football).

THE CERVICAL DISCS

The problems I have discussed so far in this chapter have pertained mostly to the discs of the lower back, the lumbar discs. However, degeneration of one or more of the cervical discs, the ones that run along the neck portion of your spine, is not an uncommon phenomenon. This is often associated with arthritic changes in the neck as well, so that there develops a combination of bony spurs plus disc protrusion which creates pressure on the spinal cord and nerve roots.

When the cervical discs are involved the symptoms are confined to the upper extremities. They usually consist of pain centered in the neck and radiating down through the shoulders and arms to the hands. If the nerve compression is excessive, the victim will develop weakness and atrophy of the forearm and hand muscles and loss of sensation in the fingers and hand.

Basically the same course of events which I have described for the lumbar region of the spine is followed in the cervical region, but there are a few significant differences between the two. One is that the neck is not subjected to the same stresses, loads, and forces that the lumbar spine is, so that cervical disc protrusions are not very large. Another is that the portion of the spinal cord that lies within the cervical region of the spinal canal is much larger and contains many more nerves. Consequently, in some respects, damage to this area can be much more serious than to the lumbar region because it involves the entire spinal cord. Except for those patients who have sudden injuries to their necks, such as cervical sprain ("whiplash" injury, a term beloved by lawyers but abhorred by all orthopedists), or a specific trauma which may lead to early or premature degeneration of a cervical disc, cervical disc problems are more common in older people than younger.

The treatment program is similar to that of lower disc-caused back pain: bed rest and cervical traction in more severe cases, cervical collars in milder cases. Occasionally surgery is required to remove a really recalcitrant disc.

Ultimately, almost all weak backs will develop disc

degeneration or herniation. If you have already been through disc treatment, you'll know how important exercise therapy is for avoiding recurrence. If you've not yet been through such treatment, but do have the kind of weak, unstable back and chronic attacks of pain and spasm I've been describing, you can be sure you're on your way to serious disc trouble. The one chance you have of cutting it off before the condition progresses to that point is to go to work on your back—now—through improved posture and exercise therapy.

SOME GOOD AND EASY BACK EXERCISES

If you have had episodes of disc-related back pain, arthritis-related back pain, or merely have a tendency to chronic strain in your back, you should be making every effort you can to strengthen your back's supporting muscles. This is desirable whether you are a weekend athlete or not. Serious back problems often strike with no apparent precipitating cause whatsoever, although by now you should realize that there is always a real underlying cause. The underlying cause is the combination of poor posture and weak musculature that leads to disc degeneration.

Serious back problems also strike those who least expect them. Many people with a love for athletics labor under the delusion that because they are active, because their bodies get exercise, their backs are impervious to spinal or muscle damage. Conventional sports activities, however, are no impediments to back degeneration. Indeed, the occasional or sporadic sports activist is probably even more susceptible to back afflictions than people who are completely sedentary.

Chronic muscle strains in the back, as a result of ordinary athletic activity, are clear signals to you that your back's muscles are not up to the task of properly supporting your spine. If you allow these strains to recur without making an attempt to forestall them, you will surely pay the piper at some later date. Since you will not want to find yourself in the position of having to give up your favorite sports, you will be well advised to embark on the brief program of back-strengthening exercises I am about to set out. These exercises are equally effective in helping you to prevent the occurrence of a serious back disorder and in preventing its recurrence if you've already been victimized.

The exercises are neither difficult nor time consuming. But don't get the idea you can breeze through them. This particular program of exercises is the one that has worked best and has had the most consistent success with all my back-pain patients. The exercises are designed to achieve two goals. One is to stretch out the tight and stiff muscles immediately around your spine and its joints in order to relieve the chronic-strain tendency that occurs as a result of their stiffness. The second is to strengthen all the muscles in your body that support your spine, so that some of the abnormal spinal loads that cause your pain will be taken up by these muscles. By strengthening those muscles, you will be simultaneously strengthening the muscles which enable you to have good posture.

Before going any further, you should observe these few basic ground rules for proper exercise:

1. *Check with your doctor to make certain that you do not have a problem that could be made worse by exercising now.* Do not start exercis-

ing until you are sure that it is all right for you
to do so.

2.   *Once you start the exercises, you must keep at
them EVERY DAY.* It is better not to start the
exercises at all unless you are willing to follow
this rule. That means every day without exception.

3.   *Avoid overdoing them at the beginning.* Overdoing them will cause undue fatigue, stiffness,
and soreness, which in turn will tempt you into
skipping days and will, in some cases, discourage you completely from giving the exercises
the chance they and you deserve.

4.   *Set aside twenty minutes a day for your daily
exercises.* Break this up into two ten-minute
periods, one after arising in the morning, the
other just before retiring at night.

All the exercises should be done on a firm surface,
preferably a carpeted floor. They should be done slowly
and carefully, with a minimum of straining.

I have divided the eight exercises into two sets of
four each. The first set consists of stretching and loosen-
ing exercises for the deeper muscles and other structures around your spine; the second consists of muscle-
strengthening exercises. You should start off with the
first four exercises alone. Once you have mastered
these and have become comfortable with them—after
two or three weeks, say—you should then proceed to
add, one at a time, the second four exercises.

With the exception of the last of the eight exercises, the standard starting position is lying flat on your
back with your knees bent and raised, the soles of your
feet on the floor, and your hands and arms flat out by
your side for easy balance. This position is very impor-

tant. By raising your knees and having your back flat against the floor, you relax all the stress and strain on your hamstring, abdominal, and lower-back muscles, as well as on your sciatic nerve. You also reduce your lumbar spinal curve.

Each exercise should be repeated five times in its entirety at the beginning. All should be done slowly, carefully and deliberately, with concentration and close attention to correct technique. Do not run through them just to get them over with. Gradually, as they become easier to do, you can add additional repetitions until you are able to accomplish ten without excessive strain. Once you have this capability, you will then be ready to go on a once-a-day maintenance program.

Exercise 1. Knee-to-Chest Raise

STEP A. From the standard starting position, pull your left knee to your chest as far as it will go without causing you pain. Hold, count slowly to five, then return your leg to the starting position.

STEP B. Repeat the same maneuver with your right leg, drawing your right knee as close as you can to your chest, holding it there for a count of five, then returning your leg to the starting position.

STEP C. Now bring both knees up toward your chest, allowing them to separate slightly so that they point toward your shoulders. When your knees are as close to your chest as you can get them, hold for a count of five, then slowly return your legs to starting position.

Run through this exercise five times to begin with, doing all three parts each time. Once you can do the entire exercise five times without difficulty, gradually increase the repetitions to ten. Do not use your arms or hands to help you in raising your knees—they are only for balance, and if you use them for leverage you will dilute the therapeutic value of the exercise. Likewise, do not strain or lunge—do the maneuvers slowly and deliberately, and always be in control of those parts of your body you are moving from one position to another.

The purpose of this exercise is to stretch out the stiff and tightened muscles, ligaments and joints of your lower back. You will find after awhile that it is very useful in relieving the constant feeling of strain and fatigue you have there.

Exercise 2. Pelvic Tilt

In this exercise you simply contract your buttocks muscles while lying in the standard starting position. Hold your buttocks clenched for a count of five, then relax them, all the time keeping your lower spine flattened against the floor. Do not try to flatten your spine by using your legs or abdominal muscles; rather, do it by concentrating on tightening the muscles of your buttocks, squeezing them together as hard as you can. You will feel your pelvis raise slightly as you do so, and the small of your back will flatten out by itself.

The purpose of this exercise is to strengthen your gluteus maximus muscles, which, when in good condition, prevent excessive lumbar spinal curve (swayback) and reduce fatigue when you stand for long periods of time.

Again, do the exercise five times to begin with, contracting your buttocks slowly, and as tightly as you can. Hold them firmly clenched for a count of five each time, with a brief rest between each repetition. Gradually work up to ten repetitions.

Exercise 3. Lateral Trunk Stretch

STEP A. This exercise is designed to stretch out the tightened muscles on either side of your spine. Start in the standard knees-raised position, but this time place your hands behind your head with your elbows flat on the floor.

STEP B. Now, cross your bent right leg over your left, just above your left knee.

STEP C. Using the weight of your right leg to force your left knee, press your left knee to the right as far as possible, preferably so that your left knee touches the floor. Hold your left knee to the floor for a count of five, then return it to the starting position and uncross your legs.

STEP D. Now reverse the process. From the same starting position, cross your left leg over your right, above the right knee.

STEP E. Using the weight of your left leg as it's crossed over the right, force your right knee to the left until it touches the floor or comes as close to it as possible. Hold there for a count of five.

STEP F. Return to the starting position, uncross your legs and, still maintaining the starting position, relax for a moment before repeating the process.

Alternate each leg five times to begin with and work gradually up to ten repetitions for each side. Again, do the exercise slowly and deliberately, without any cheating or short-cutting. If you are at first unable to get either or both knees to the floor without excessive strain on your back and limbs, try to get them as close to the floor as possible and keep working at it until you are able to touch the floor with your knees. At all times keep your upper back flat on the floor, using your elbows to achieve this balance. As you master this very valuable exercise you will feel the muscles in either side of your torso stretch with each alternating maneuver.

Exercise 4.   Single Straight-Leg Raise

STEP A. From the standard starting position, straighten out your left leg and press it flat against the floor with your left knee rigid. Then, as slowly as you can, and without using your hands and arms for leverage, raise the straightened leg as high as you can, until you get pain or excessive tightness in your thigh. When you've raised the leg as high as you can, hold for a count of five. Then, still as slowly and deliberately as you can, let your leg drop back to the floor, keeping your knee straight. Relax for a moment, then repeat for a total of five consecutive repetitions.

STEP B. When your left leg is back on the floor after the last repetition, return to the standard starting position. Then straighten out your right leg and repeat the exercise, slowly raising your straightened leg as high as you can, holding for a count of five, and slowly returning it to the floor. Again, repeat for a total of five consecutive repetitions.

When doing this exercise, never swing your legs up and do not use your hands to help you push. Keep your lower back flat on the floor as you raise each straightened leg, and constantly strive to raise each leg as high as you can, working gradually over a period of time up to ten consecutive repetitions for each leg.

This is another valuable exercise for stretching and strengthening your tight hamstring, buttocks, and hip muscles, which go a long way toward preserving and supporting your lower back.

After you have mastered the first four exercises and can do each of them ten times comfortably, you are ready to go on to the second set of four, which begins with Exercise 5. Whereas the first four are designed mainly to aid you in *stretching out* the supporting structures of your back, the second four are intended to *strengthen* the important muscles that keep your spine in proper balance and configuration.

Exercise 5. Half Sit-Ups

STEP A. Again, starting from the standard position, slowly raise your head and neck until your chin touches the top of your chest.

STEP B. As you maintain this position, and without raising your mid- or lower back off the floor, reach both hands forward and place them on the tops of both your knees, which are bent. Hold this position for a count of five.

STEP C. After you've counted to five, slowly return to the starting position, relax for a moment, then repeat.

This exercise, like the others, should be done five times to begin with and gradually increased to ten repetitions. It strengthens your abdominal and lower-back muscles, doing the work of conventional sit-ups without causing the back strain such sit-ups often produce. As with all the other exercises in this program, it is important that it be done slowly, deliberately, and with concentration. As your abdominal muscles become strengthened, they will better be able to provide the frontal support your back requires, the lack of which is so often a contributing factor in back pain.

Exercise 6. Nose-to-Knee Touch

STEP A. From the standard starting position, bring your left knee slowly to your chest, as in Exercise 1. As you clasp it tightly against your chest with both hands, extend and straighten your right leg until it is flat on the floor.

STEP B. Keeping your lower back flat on the floor, raise your head and bring it forward until you can touch your nose to your bent knee. Hold your nose against your knee for a count of five.

STEP C. Slowly drop your head back to the floor. Relax for a moment, still keeping your left knee clamped to your chest, then raise your head and touch your nose to your knee again.

Do this exercise five times with your left knee raised to your chest, then switch and do it five times with your right knee raised. This exercise strengthens your abdominal muscles and at the same time stretches the opposite hip flexors.

Exercise 7. Scissors

STEP A. This is a standard exercise used in most calisthenic programs for the abdominal, hip, and back muscles. I would like you to do it this way. Start again from the standard position, bring both knees to your chest, and hold there for a moment while you concentrate on keeping good balance with your back flat on the floor.

STEP B. Using your hands to balance yourself, straighten both legs into the air together.

STEP C. With your legs straight and extended vertically, very slowly scissor them front-to-back ten times, opening the scissors as wide as you can each time while maintaining good control and balance.

STEP D. Once you've completed the front-to-back scissor, proceed to scissor your legs laterally, or crossways, ten more times, alternating right leg over left, right leg under left.

STEP E. On the completion of the lateral scissors, return to the starting position, first by slowly bringing your knees down to your chest, then by returning your feet to the floor.

Relax for a few moments, then repeat the exercise again. This exercise will further stretch out and strengthen your hamstring, lower-back, and hip muscles, and will also strengthen your abdominal muscles.

Exercise 8. Hip Hyperextension

STEP A. For this exercise you turn over onto your stomach. Lie flat and let your hands and arms fall naturally above your shoulders.

STEP B. Stiffen your left leg, making sure your knee is as rigid as you can make it, then slowly raise your stiffened leg from the hip. Do not rotate your pelvis in order to get your leg off the floor—keep it flat. Raise and lower your left leg five times consecutively.

STEP C. Return to the starting position, relax for a moment, then stiffen your right leg and repeat the exercise five times.

Initially you may find it very difficult to lift your legs off the floor at all. Do not despair, and do not cheat; it will come if you work at it. If all you are able to do at first is tighten up your buttocks and leg muscles and get your leg off just slightly, that's fine. Starting with five repetitions for each leg, work up to ten. When you are able to lift each leg between ten and fifteen degrees off the floor ten consecutive times without undue strain, you will have reached your goal for this exercise. The exercise stretches and strengthens your hip muscles and at the same time further strengthens your buttocks and lower-back muscles.

In doing Exercises 5 through 8 you should start with 5, do it for a few days until it becomes comfortable, then add 6. Do 6 for a few days, then add 7, and finally 8. It should take you between two and three weeks before you are doing all eight exercises. Stick with your twice-a-day schedule for another two to three weeks, or until you have mastered each exercise and your back pain has subsided.

Once this occurs you can go on a maintenance schedule of once a day, but keep to that schedule faithfully. Don't think that once your pain and stiffness have subsided you can do without the exercises. If you continue to do them, you will then be able to go out and resume your normal physical activities—even sports— without fear of your back pain recurring. If you stop doing them, your pain will sooner or later return, and you'll be back where you started.

I have deliberately kept this therapeutic exercise program limited to eight exercises. I have found from experience that when there are too many exercises, none of them get done. This combination of exercises has proved to be the most successful with my patients, and it takes no more than fifteen to twenty minutes a day to accomplish it. It is certainly worth it to devote this small amount of time to ensuring yourself a healthy back, free of pain and instability.

7

YOUR ANKLE MISERIES

The ankle is easily the fourth most troublesome site in the body when it comes to athletics. The ankle is not only the area that bears the most body weight, it is also one of the more complex and delicate joints in the body. We saw earlier the basic construction of the joint itself insofar as the bones are concerned, but what we saw only scratched the surface. Indeed, the ankle is so complicated a mechanism that it's a wonder it doesn't lead the list as the source of sports-related ailments.

The reason it doesn't is precisely because of its complexity. Because it has so many tasks to perform, nature has provided it with more supporting and bracing parts than any other joint in the body. If you were able to look inside your ankle—above and below the joint itself—you would see an incredible maze of ligaments, tendons, bones, and muscle attachments packed into a small area. It is these tissues that give the joint both its mobility and its support, and provide it with its relatively low affliction rate in the face of the high rate of stress it must constantly bear.

However, the ankle *is* prone to a few common chronic ailments, most of which arise out of sudden injuries, and it is worth your while to know something more about them and about how they can be prevented or managed.

The ankle is, as I have said, a hinge-type saddle joint—that is, a joint in which the bones articulate with one another in a way similar to the way a horseback rider moves in relationship to the saddle. The joint itself is formed by the lower ends of the two lower-leg bones, the tibia and the fibula, and the upper end of the ankle bone, the talus. This bone is connected in front and behind to the bones of the upper foot and heel, and acts not only in the function of the ankle but of the foot as well.

Enveloping the joint—that is, around the articulating surfaces of the talus, tibia, and fibula—is the standard synovial membrane, which, as with the knee and other joints, lubricates and nourishes the cartilage covering the articular surfaces. Covering this is the capsule, a dense, fibrous tissue which both protects the synovium and helps to hold the joint together.

But what holds the joint together most effectively is an intricate series of ligaments which connect the three bones of the joint to each other and to the many bones of the foot below. Since there are over a dozen separate bones in the foot, you can see the reason for the existence of so many ligaments around the ankle. Most ankle miseries occur in two of these ligaments.

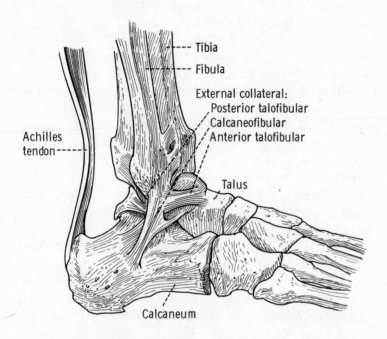

FIG. 12. *A skeletal view of your ankle from the lateral, or outer, aspect, showing the three branches of the external, or lateral, collateral ligament. The* anterior talofibular *branch is the one most often subject to ankle miseries.*

On the outer side of the ankle is a ligament that is akin to the knee's lateral collateral ligament. It is the major ligament supporting the outer side of the ankle and acts as a checkrein, preventing the joint from bending excessively inward, when we put our full weight on it. Although it is generally referred to as the external, or lateral collateral, ligament of the ankle, it has three branches, each of which has a separate function while still acting in concert with the other two to provide lateral support and bracing.

The ligament originates at the outer side of the fibula, which is the outer of the two lower-leg bones which form part of the ankle joint. Its exact site of origin is the *lateral malleolus*—the large knob you can feel on the outer surface of your ankle. From there it divides and travels in three different directions: anteriorly, or forward; posteriorly, or rearward; and inferiorly, or downward.

The latter two branches are called the *posterior* and *inferior calcaneo-fibular* ligaments. This is because they connect the fibular portion of the ankle joint to the heel bone, which is known as the *calcaneum*.

It is the other branch that we are most concerned with, the anterior branch, because it directly connects two of the three bones of the ankle joint itself—the fibula above to the talus below. This short branch is called the *anterior talo-fibular ligament*. It is the ligament most often involved in ankle ailments.

On the inner, or medial, side of the ankle is the lateral collateral ligament's opposite number, the *medial collateral ligament*. It is also known as the *talo-tibial* ligament because it connects the tibia, or inner lower-leg bone, to the talus, or ankle bone. But I shall call it by its most common name, the *medial deltoid ligament*. Its exact site of origin is the *medial malleolus* —the large knob you can feel on the inner aspect of your ankle.

This ligament is called "deltoid" because it is wide and fan shaped. It is a continuous band of tissue and is not separated like the lateral collateral ligament. However, it not only connects the tibia to the talus but also, due to its wide dimension, has a connection to the heel bone as well. The main function of the medial deltoid ligament is to prevent the ankle from turning excessively inward, and the foot outward, when we put our full weight on it.

These two ligaments—the *anterior talofibular* on the outer side and the *medial deltoid* on the inner—are the chief villains in the chronic condition known as "weak ankles."

WEAK ANKLES, OR SKATER'S ANKLES

Weak or collapsing ankles can plague one in just about any sport, but it is in ice-skating that it is most infuriating. Yet it is not just the two crucial side-supporting ligaments that account for such a condition. The ankles are also supported and moved by muscles around the joints, and when these are weak the result will show in a tendency of the ankles to bend excessively from side to side.

Weak ankles can be congenital—that is, one can be born with thin or weak ankle muscles. Or, one or both strong ankles can evolve into weak ankles through injury and chronic trauma. In these instances, the injuries are usually suffered during childhood, and the condition is carried into adult life. In either case, the condition can be overcome by understanding the role of the relevant ligaments and muscles and working to strengthen them.

Most incapacitating ankle injuries, especially when there are no bone fractures involved, take the form of severe sprains. They result from episodes in which a great and sudden stress is applied to the anterior talofibular ligament (on the outer aspect of the ankle) or to the medial deltoid ligament (on the inner aspect) through a turning-in or -out of the side of the foot when it strikes the ground. Such episodes generally occur when the foot strikes an uneven surface during walking or running, or when it strikes the ground already turned in or out, as when jumping. In either case, the weight of the body is concentrated in the affected ligament, and, as the force overpowers the ligament's maximum checkrein capability, the ligament tears—either partially or wholly.

Complete tears, or ruptures, of the ankles' side-supporting ligaments generally require surgery to restore proper ankle function. But since these come under the category of injuries rather than ailments, we are more interested in partial tears. Partial tears are the most frequent *underlying causes* of weak ankles. When the checkrein function of the damaged ligaments is not reinforced by a strengthening of the supporting muscles, this becomes the *precipitating cause*.

Because most severe ankle sprains come about through the foot turning inward under the ankle, it is the anterior talo-fibular ligament that is most often damaged and weakened. What follows is a chronic tendency of the ankle to collapse inward whenever the foot strikes an uneven surface. Yet, although outward sprains are not as common, when they do occur—that is, when the medial deltoid ligament is damaged—the same principles apply. However, the deltoid is an extremely strong ligament; often, instead of tearing, it will simply pull off a piece of bone from the talus.

So, then, if one or both of your ankles have a tendency to sprain repeatedly, it is probably due to the fact that one or both of your anterior talo-fibular ligaments have been damaged through earlier injury. Each time you further sprain your ankle you will compromise the ligament's checkrein function a bit more, and eventually your ankle will grow so weak that it will become a hazard in many of your favorite sports.

Of course, taping your ankle, or wearing a brace, can help provide stability. But these devices are cumbersome and tend to slow you down. Moreover, they encourage the further weakening of the muscles that support the ankle. The real answer to your problem is the restoration of muscle strength through therapeutic exercises.

I'm not going to get into the names of all the muscles that support and move the ankle. Suffice it to say that some originate in the lower leg (the *gastrocnemius*, which also plays a role in knee flexion, you'll remember, is one of these) and connect through tendons below the ankle joint and in the foot, and some originate in the foot and connect above the joint. By doing a few simple exercises over a period of time, you will strengthen your ankle muscles and take some of the burden for the ankles' support off your ligaments.

Exercise 1. Foot Eversion

When your anterior talo-fibular ligament is torn or otherwise strained, you will have pain and swelling across the outer aspects of your ankle. This means also that your lateral ankle muscles—known as the *peroneal* muscles—are weak. They can be best strengthened with this isometric exercise. It is advisable to do the exercise with both feet at once.

Sit on a chair with both feet flat on the floor, or lie down with the feet flat against a wall. Then evert your feet while keeping them pressed against the surface— that is, slowly raise the outer margins of your feet so that your ankle bends inward. Raise them as high as you can, keeping the inner margins against the surface, and hold for a count of five. Relax and repeat for ten repetitions, then gradually increase the repetitions over a period of time until you can do fifty without overly fatiguing the peroneal muscles.

After you can achieve fifty repetitions comfortably, you should graduate to performing the exercise against resistance or with weights strapped to your feet. Additional strengthening can be obtained by walking with your feet everted—that is, with their outer margins deliberately raised.

Exercise 2.   Foot Inversion

This is generally the same exercise for the muscles that support the inner aspect of your ankles. Instead of raising the outer margins of your feet, raise the inner margins. Otherwise do everything the same.

Actually, even though ailments involving the inner aspects of the ankle, or the medial deltoid ligament, are not anywhere near as common as those affecting the lateral, or anterior talo-fibular, ligament, you should do both of the above exercises with equal energy and devotion. This is because they work on all the muscles, inner and outer, along the sides of your ankles and are highly effective, when performed together, in overcoming chronic weak ankles—the bane not only of skaters and skiers but of tennis players and other sports enthusiasts as well.

And speaking of skiers, this brings us to another ailment of the ankle which, although it can appear in any "sudden-stop-and-start" sport, seems to be mushrooming in incidence along with rapid rise in skiing interest.

SKIER'S HEEL

When we think of the ankle we usually tend to think of its inner and outer aspects, as in ankle sprains. But in recent years, as a result of the skiing boom, we've come to learn that the ankle has another important dimension: its backside, so to speak. I'm talking, of course, about what is called in formal anatomy the *tendo calcaneus,* in general medicine the *Achilles tendon,* and in lay circles the *Achilles heel.* Since distress in this area most often occurs in skiers, it is fast becoming known as "skier's heel."

The *tendo calcaneus,* or *Achilles tendon,* is the long, thick, rounded tendon which you can feel at the back of your ankle and which attaches the muscles in the rear of the calf to the calcaneum, or heel bone. These muscles—the *gastrocnemius,* which I've already described as being a flexor of the knee, and the *soleus,* which along with the gastrocnemius is the principal *flexor* of the ankle—share the Achilles tendon in common. Like the flexor and extensor tendons in the elbow, the Achilles tendon can be strained and become inflamed as a result of repeated overloads. Unlike the extensor tendon in the elbow, though, because it is such a long tendon it also has a frequent tendency to tear, or rupture. It is for this reason it is called the Achilles tendon—after the hero of Homer's *Iliad,* the great warrior of the Trojan war whose only weakness manifested itself when his *tendo calcaneus* was cut.

Modern-day ruptures of the tendon occur fre-

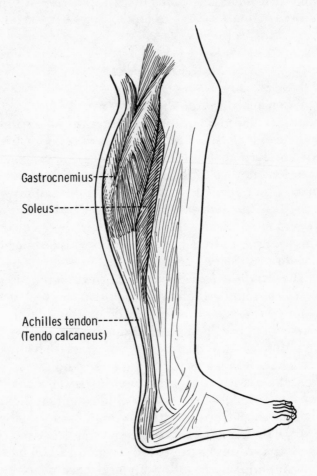

Gastrocnemius

Soleus

Achilles tendon
(Tendo calcaneus)

FIG. 13. *The Achilles tendon and the muscles it connects to your heel bone.*

quently, as I have said, among skiing enthusiasts. Such ruptures have a combination of precipitating and underlying causes. The most obvious are the strains and stresses placed on the tendon during a day of skiing. In no other sport is the Achilles tendon required to endure such continual overloads.

Corollary causes are the nature of the principal maneuvers of skiing and the design and construction of the ski boot.

The principal maneuver of skiing is the turn. In order to make a turn—whether snowplow, stem, or parallel—the skier must abruptly jerk his heels upward, then down again. At the same time, the boot is constructed in such a way that the forepart of the foot is virtually immobilized. Thus, the forces and stresses of the constant movement of the lower limbs in skiing are not distributed throughout the foot as they are in other sports. Rather, they are concentrated, and terminate, in the ankle. But the ankle, too, is bound tightly into the boot by virtue of its design—at least in its lateral aspects. The only part of the ankle really free to move is the part that permits us to raise and lower the heel. That part, of course, is the Achilles tendon. Therefore, most of the forces are concentrated in, and terminate, there.

One final underlying cause of skier's heel is weak or unconditioned calf muscles, especially the muscles that attach to the Achilles tendon and enable it to raise the heel. Just as many of the cases of tennis elbow I treat are associated with underdeveloped forearms, so too are many of the cases of Achilles-tendon rupture I treat associated with flabby or underdeveloped calf muscles.

Put all these causes together—and add to them the fatigue factor on the Achilles tendon and calf muscles which accrues from hours of repeated and constant strains of turning, edging, and trying to keep one's skis parallel—and you have an ideal set of conditions for the rupture, or at the very best the partial tear and/or inflammation, of the Achilles tendon.

When an Achilles tendon ruptures, you'll know it immediately. You will not be able to raise your heel, will find yourself in great pain, and will only be able to walk by dragging your heel behind you. Such an injury calls for immediate treatment, for although tendon tissue heals when it is partially torn, when it is totally torn, or ruptured, it will only heal in the slack position. Hence you will always walk with "heel-drag."

Surgery is relatively simple. The tendon is restored to its normal tautness. Any gap is bridged with tissue borrowed from elsewhere in the area and sutured into the damaged tendon. After a period of recuperation, the repaired tendon returns to normal, or almost normal, function. I have also treated complete tendon rupture through simple cast immobilization for eight or ten weeks, and have had good results.

Ruptured Achilles tendon can occur suddenly or gradually. No matter how it occurs—except in cases of sudden, extremely excessive overloads—it is usually preceded by partial tearing and/or Achilles tendinitis. Thus, in many instances the victim will be forewarned. If he or she heeds the warning, more serious damage will be avoided.

Partial tears will create pain and a reduced heel-raising capability. About the only viable treatment for such tears is a period of rest to give the torn fibers a chance to heal, then a program of exercises to strengthen the calf muscles.

Achilles tendinitis also creates pain at the site of attachment of tendon to muscle. This condition, again, is caused by excessive strain on the calf muscle, but the symptoms are significantly different. As in tennis elbow, when there is continual strain on the tendon attachments, the tendon and muscle contract in a kind of permanent spasmodic reaction. This contraction forces the heel to raise involuntarily, and any attempt to lower it will merely exacerbate the pain.

Again, rest is the prescription here, and perhaps an injection of cortisone to relieve the pain and inflammation, followed by special exercises to stretch the tendon and build up the calf muscles.

SOME SIMPLE
ACHILLES TENDON EXERCISES

Whether you have already had Achilles-tendon ailments or not, if your sport is skiing, tennis, or any other activity that exerts excessive strains on your tendon— and especially if your calf muscles are on the weak or underdeveloped side in relation to the rest of your physique—you should do at least two exercises designed to build-up your muscles and make your Achilles tendon more supple.

Exercise 1. Heel Dip-and-Raise
Stand, bracing yourself, on the balls of your feet at the edge of a step so that your heels hang well out over the edge. Lower your heels as far as you can, then slowly raise them up by standing on the tips of your toes. Hold the tiptoe position for a count of five, then repeat. Start with ten repetitions and work gradually up to fifty. This exercise will stretch your Achilles tendon and strengthen your calf muscles.

Exercise 2. Wall Bounce
Stand well away from a wall, facing it, with your feet flat on the floor. Then, keeping your legs and body

straight, feet still flat, fall towards the wall and catch yourself with your hands. With your feet still flat on the floor, commence to bounce back and forth against the wall, using your arms both to push away and to prevent you from hitting it with your shoulders and head. This exercise will stretch out your Achilles tendons and, if done regularly, provide them with maximum pliability.

Another beneficial routine to get into—one you can do anywhere, anytime—is occasionally to walk a few blocks with pronounced, deliberate heel-raising motion of your ankles. In other words, on the way to the subway, movies, or wherever, concentrate on completing each step you take with an exaggerated tiptoe flourish, bouncing off the balls of your feet as you stride into the next step.

After a block or so of walking in this style you will clearly feel the benefits in your calf muscles. The combination of these three routines will definitely enhance your Achilles tendons' ability to withstand stress and fatigue without tearing or becoming inflamed—another potential misery down the drain!

8

YOUR SHOULDER MISERIES

"Put your shoulder into it!" "Learn to shoulder your
responsibilities!" "I'm carrying the world on my shoulders."

These familiar phrases are indicative of how we
think of the shoulder: strong, weight-supporting, reliable. Generally speaking, the first and last images are
usually accurate—the human shoulder *is* strong and
reliable. The second characterization, though—that the
shoulder is weight-supporting—is slightly inaccurate
and leads to some of the misconceptions about the
shoulder which are responsible for getting it into trouble.

The shoulder, one of the largest joints of the body,
is not, in man, a weight-bearing mechanism, and it is
this fact that accounts for its unique design and mobil-

ity. It is because it is not weight-bearing that it is capable of its wide range of motion. Yet ironically, its wide range of motion, plus the fact that it is not designed to bear great weight, account for most of the ailments it develops—even though they are relatively few compared to the other major joints of the body.

The shoulder is a ball-and-socket joint capable of motion in almost every direction, and capable also of full rotation. Thanks to the design of our shoulder joints we are able to engage in a wide variety of sports. Without our shoulders' mobility we would find most popular sports impossible to play. Thus, when their natural mobility is hampered or restricted by injury, inflammation, and pain, we usually are forced to take a sabbatical from our favorite athletic activities.

Fortunately, as I have suggested, the shoulder suffers fewer chronic athletic ailments than most other regions of the body. Those that occur usually do so because their owners fail to understand that their shoulders were not designed to bear great weight stresses—either sudden or gradual ones. Our shoulders are so marvelously free that we tend to think they are capable of anything. Indeed they are—almost. To understand the exception is to understand how to prevent or avoid shoulder miseries!

THE BASIC ANATOMY OF THE SHOULDER

The shoulder joint is formed by the conjunction of two bones: the upper-arm bone, or humerus, and a large, flat bone often called the "wing bone" but anatomically named the *scapula*. This bone has three projections—a spine on its back aspect, a curved rim along the top, and a half-socket on its outer aspect. The upper end of the humerus is rounded into a ball shape and projects inward and upward toward the scapula at an angle. This ball-shape projection, known as the "head" of the humerus, fits loosely into the corresponding half-socket at the side and top of the scapula. The socket is formed by a concave depression in the scapula itself, called the *glenoid cavity*. A projection of the scapula overlaps the entire joint and is called the *acromion* (commonly known as the "shoulder cap").

The scapula itself is attached to the rest of the skeleton by muscles, but its acromion is attached directly to the *clavicle*, or collar bone, which in turn crosses the base of your throat to attach to the *sternum*, or breastbone.

So, then, we have the head of the humerus, ball-shaped, articulating with the half-socket, or glenoid, side of the scapula. Notice that I don't say the head of the humerus lies *in* the socket. It doesn't. In the first place, the socket is not that deep, and it doesn't really cover the head of the humerus. If it did—that is, if the head of the humerus was buried deep in the socket—we would have much less motion in our arm than we have.

Second, since the shoulder was not designed to be a weight-bearing joint, it does not require the bony stability that a weight-bearing, ball-and-socket joint, such as the hips, needs. Thus, the juxtaposition and articulation of the bones in the shoulder may be termed "loose" as compared to those in the hips and other joints, which are "tight." With the exception of this difference, *and two others*, the construction of the shoulder joint is the same as that of all the other joints. The joint itself is enveloped by the usual synovial cap-

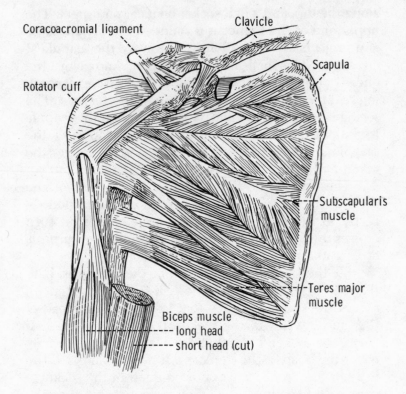

FIG. 14. *A frontal view of your shoulder, showing the muscles, bones, tendons, and ligaments most susceptible to injury in weekend sports.*

sule and is blanketed by muscles, tendons, and ligaments which both move and support it. Here lies *one* of the other two differences I mentioned.

Because the shoulder is a "loose" joint, the ligaments which connect the bones to one another are necessarily looser and more slack than in the other joints of the body. The result of this is that shoulder ailments very seldom involve the ligaments. Except in severe shoulder-separation injuries due to extremely excessive forces, the shoulder ligaments generally remain out of harm's way.

This, however, accounts for the *other* major difference. Because of the natural laxity of the ligaments, it falls to the muscles of the shoulder, *and their tendons,* to support and stabilize the joint. Therefore the tendons of the shoulder are largely subject to injury and chronic ailment.

This leads to what can be considered a third difference—a difference which accounts for the large majority of annoying and painful shoulder ailments, not counting, of course, separations and dislocations.* This ailment is commonly called "thrower's" or "tennis shoulder," and I shall get to it in a page or two. Before discussing it, however, it is important that we understand in more detail the role of the muscles and tendons of the shoulder.

Since the shoulder possesses mobility in many directions, many more muscles are required to move and support it than other joints. As a result, the area of the shoulder is jam-packed with muscles and tendons that

---

*Shoulder separations and dislocations are injuries that do not really fall within the purview of this book. However, they deserve a mention, especially because so many people do not know the difference between the two.

A *shoulder dislocation* is an injury in which the head of the humerus is actually separated from its socket. It is usually brought about by great stresses on the arm, and most often occurs among football tacklers. It is painful, but not serious. However, due to damage to the ligaments, tendons, and lubricating components, it can produce chronic instability.

A *shoulder separation* is also an injury, but not to the shoulder joint itself. Rather, it involves the articular junction of the acromion (shoulder cap) and the clavicle just above the shoulder joint (see illustration). It is usually brought about by falls onto the shoulder under heavy weight, causing the two bones to become displaced in relation to one another. It is extremely painful, and the recuperation time, with the arm and shoulder trussed and immobilized, can last as long as eight weeks.

crisscross, intertwine, overlap, and interact. No single muscle group has only one function; they all act in concert, some coming into play more strenuously than others, depending on the precise direction of the movement.

To detail all these muscles by name and function would be much too complicating for our purposes. Suffice it to say that some are located across the top of the chest, others along the top of the shoulder, others in the back and around the ribs, and still others in the arm. There are, however, three special muscles and associated tendons that *are* important for our purpose because they play a signal role in most ordinary shoulder miseries.

These muscle groups are the *biceps* muscles of the arm, the four muscles that form what is known as the *"rotator cuff"* of the shoulder, and the *deltoid* muscle.

Every time we flex our shoulder or move it and our arm forward, we do so principally with the biceps muscles of our upper arm and the front portions of the deltoid muscle. Every time we rotate our shoulder outward or externally, we do so principally with three of the muscles that constitute the rotator cuff and hold the humerus to the scapula. When we rotate our shoulder inward, the fourth rotator-cuff muscle—the *subscapularis*—comes into play. Throwing sports, tennis stroking, swimming, and skiing are just four of the many athletic activities that involve forward motion and inward and outward rotation of the arm and shoulder. And it is these in which the most common ailment of the shoulder—"thrower's shoulder"—develops.

THROWER'S SHOULDER

Thrower's shoulder is really a tendinitis of the shoulder. It occurs mostly as an inflammation of either the tendon that connects the biceps muscle of the upper arm to the scapula of the shoulder, or of the tendon that connects the muscles of the shoulder's rotator cuff to the humerus of the arm. Let's have a closer look at these tendons.

You'll recall that I said a page-or-so ago that in addition to the looseness of the shoulder's articulation and the natural laxity of its ligaments, there is a third difference between the shoulder joint and other joints of the body, and that this difference involves the tendons. More specifically, the difference lies in the biceps tendon, which attaches the upper-arm muscle to the scapula.

You know by now that in order to move a joint, the muscles that do so must cross the joint—that is, if they originate from below or above a joint, they must extend and connect beyond it in a direction opposite to their site of origin. You've learned, for instance, that the extensor muscles of the elbow originate in the forearm and cross the elbow to attach to the lateral epicondyle of the humerus. The attaching device is, of course, the extensor tendon. You've also learned that the quadriceps muscles originate in the thigh and cross the knee, through their attachment to the kneecap, to connect to the bone below the knee. In this case, the attaching device is known as the quadriceps tendon. In both cases the muscles, by being so-attached, provide their respective joints with specific kinds of motion.

So, too, with the biceps muscles of the upper arm in relation to the shoulder. In order to move the shoulder forward, they must attach on the far side of the joint, which they do. It is the way in which they do that is exceptional, and that also provides dangers for their connecting biceps tendon.

The biceps muscles originate in the front of the upper arm and flow to both the elbow and the shoulder. One would ordinarily think they would attach to the far side of the shoulder joint in the conventional way—that they would travel up over the rounded head of the humerus, cross the forward aspect of the joint, and attach to the top of the scapula's socket.

But because the area over the forward aspect of the joint is so crowded a maze of muscles coming from the chest, the top of the shoulder, and the back, such is not the case. There is simply no room for the biceps muscle to cross *over* the joint here, so nature devised an ingenious alternative. It routed the biceps muscles or, to be more accurate, the biceps tendon, directly through the shoulder joint! By so doing, nature solved a space problem. But it also *created* a problem, which neatly illustrates the old axiom that you never gain something without losing something in return.

In no other joint of the body does a tendon actually enter and exit the joint itself. The biceps tendon enters the joint through a groove at the top of the humerus. It pierces the synovial capsule, lies free within the joint, and then exits to attach to the upper rim of the scapula's socket.

Because of its unique position and its role in one of the primary motions of the arm and shoulder, the biceps tendon is subject to considerably more strain than most other tendons of the shoulder. The strain usually occurs when throwing an object while off balance, when serving incorrectly in tennis, when rotating the arm and shoulder forward in a hard swimming stroke, and when performing rapid poling motions during skiing, as in the *wedeln*. In each case, either excessive weight (skiing) or excessive force (throwing, tennis, swimming) is placed on the biceps tendon at its moment of optimal stretch through the fore-rotating motion of the shoulder.

Repeated irritation of that portion of the tendon that lies in the groove causes inflamation and pain. *Biceps tendinitis* follows, with pain in front of the shoulder radiating into the arm. All of you who have or have had the condition know well how infuriating it can be.

As in all tendon ailments, rest is the first stage of treatment, followed possibly by an injection of cortisone to relieve any residual pain and promote healing. But again, as in most breakdowns of joint-connecting tissues, the tears and inflammations occur because the supporting and attaching muscles are not strong enough to withstand the abnormal stresses placed on the joints. So, to ensure that the condition does not become chronic, it is necessary to strengthen the muscles around the site of the biceps tendon. This can be done easily enough with the three general, all-purpose shoulder exercises I shall outline at the end of this chapter.

SHOULDER BURSITIS

The other ailment of the shoulder which comes under the heading of "thrower's shoulder" is the impingement of the rotator cuff against the *coraco-*

acromial ligament, which causes a general condition of *bursitis* to develop in the shoulder. Chronic bursitis is often a byproduct of tendinitis.

The rotator cuff of the shoulder, as the term implies, controls and stabilizes the rotation of the shoulder as it rotates through its various stages. The rotator cuff

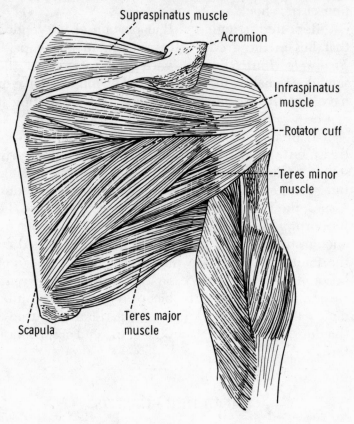

FIG. 15. *A rear view of your shoulder. Note the muscles of the rotator cuff.*

consists of four muscles which attach to the upper end of the humerus and control shoulder rotation.

One large, single muscle originates along the front surface of the scapula. It crosses the front of the shoulder joint and attaches to the inner surface of the humerus just below its head. It is called the *subscapularis* muscle.

Coming from the top and rear surfaces of the scapula is a group of three mixed and layered muscles that cross the top and rear aspects of the joint and attach, through a common tendon, to the lateral side of the humerus, just below the head. These three muscles are called the *supraspinatus,* the *infraspinatus,* and the *teres minor.* They are the muscles that form the rotator cuff.

The *supraspinatus* muscle originates along the top of the scapula; the *infraspinatus* from the rear of the scapula in the region of the shoulder blade; and the *teres minor* from the outer margin of the scapula. Now I know this might be getting a bit complicated, but hang on for a moment because there's just one more thing you really need to know to understand how bursitis develops in the shoulder.

We already know that the shoulder joint itself is inherently loose. The muscles of the rotator cuff, however, serve to keep it from being too loose—they wrap over and around the joint and hold the rounded head of the humerus firm against the half-socket of the scapula. Nevertheless, a partial separation of the joint can easily be demonstrated by X rays when someone hangs by the arm from a pole. What happens here is that the supraspinatus muscle of the rotator cuff—the

muscle that passes over the top of the shoulder joint—
retracts the head of the humerus slightly upward. The
joint subluxates—that is, the two opposed bones become slightly displaced under the stress of hanging, and
the joint opens up abnormally.

Now imagine that you are not hanging by your arm
but are trying to throw a football fifty yards, or trying
to *wedeln* down a steep ski slope, or trying to hit a
tennis serve with all your power in an effort to ace your
opponent. It is at the moment when your shoulder is in
the extreme top of its rotation that you release the
pigskin or plant the ski pole or thwack the tennis ball,
at which time the greatest stress is applied to your
rotator-cuff muscles—especially the supraspinatus. The
moment is akin to hanging by your arm, although the
force on your supraspinatus muscle is greater and more
sudden. The muscle pulls on your humerus, allowing
your joint to subluxate for a split second and the head
of your humerus to slide upward against its socket. Such
an abnormal joint motion will create a strain not only
on your biceps tendon inside the joint but even more
significantly on the bones' articulating surfaces and on
the lubricating bursae within and around the joint capsule.

Repeated and recurrent stresses of this type, with
the joint opening up in such a manner, will cause the
bursae to become irritated and inflamed. The result is
bursitis of the shoulder.

This is not the only way bursitis occurs in the shoulder, but it is the most common among weekend athletes. Indeed, any abnormal motion in the joint can lead
to bursitis. Most abnormal motions, unless they are
brought about by injury, develop as a result, again, of
weak muscles. When a certain maneuver produces a
stress on the supporting ligaments and tendons around

the joint, other muscles must be trained to absorb the strain and retain the articular integrity of the joint.

Treatment of bursitis follows the same formula for most cases of inflamed body tissue: first, rest, followed by cortisone, if necessary. Heat treatments might also help. But the main thing, once the pain and stiffness are relieved, is to go to work on those shoulder muscles to prevent the onset of chronic bursitis, which is difficult to overcome without surgery.

THREE ALL-PURPOSE SHOULDER EXERCISES

Of course, exercise is not the only answer. You must also revise the bad throwing, stroking, or poling habits you have developed. But these three exercises should go a long way toward making up for the excessive shoulder stresses that result from your faulty athletic techniques.

Exercise 1. *Arm-and-Shoulder Pendulum*

Bend at the waist ninety degrees with your legs slightly spread. Brace your free hand on your opposite knee. Swing your other arm in a wide arc across your body from right to left in a pendulum motion. Bring your arm as high as you can to the right, let it swing down toward the floor and across your knees, then up to the left as far as it will go. If it is not painful, take a five-pound dumbbell or a heavy book and repeat the exercise. Work up to fifty repetitions from twenty, then increase the weight by two pounds and begin again at twenty. This exercise stretches and strengthens all the muscles around the front of the shoulder joint.

Exercise 2.   Side-and-Front Arm Raise

Stand erect. Lift your stiffened arm slowly to a horizontal plane in front of your body. Hold for a slow count of five. Then move it slowly on the same horizontal plane to the side of your body. Hold for another slow count of five. Then lower the arm to your side again, slowly. Thirty repetitions.

Start this exercise holding a two-pound weight if you are a man, one-pound if a woman. Men can progress to ten pounds in two-pound increments; women to five pounds in one-pound increments. With each increase of weight, work back up to thirty repetitions.

Exercise 3.   Doorway Isometric

(A) Stand in a conventional doorway with your feet together. With your arms straight, press the backs of both hands against the frame as though you were trying to expand it. Press hard for a slow count of five, then relax. Repeat for thirty repetitions. When you can do thirty easily, increase the counterpressure by holding for longer counts.

(B) Do the same exercise, except this time do it from above. That is, raise your arms straight over your head and then press the backs of both hands against the side frame from above. You may alternate the two exercises.

LITTLE-LEAGUE SHOULDER

There are a number of other ailments of the shoulder in the weekend athlete, but these follow approximately the same patterns that bring about tendinitis and bursitis—that is, they involve other muscles, tendons, and, sometimes, ligaments of the shoulder. But there is one ailment that involves bone, and although it is usually limited to children, it is worth looking at briefly because, in their way, many children are weekend athletes and the ailment can carry over and cause a variety of problems in adulthood. The technical name for this ailment is *osteochondrosis of the proximal humeral epiphysis,* but it is more commonly known as "little-league shoulder."

Up until the adolescent stage of our development, the growth of our musculo-skeletal system is incomplete. Our bones, especially at the joints, must have the ability to expand with the rest of our growth. As a result, the ends of the bones have sectors called "growth plates."

The growth plates are usually immune from damage in normal childhood and preadolescent activities. But in certain sports the growth plates of youngsters can be damaged by excessive and recurrent stresses on these areas. This holds especially true for the shoulder and elbow growth-plates of the humerus in throwing sports, of which baseball is the most popular. And with the rise of the little-league phenomenon over the past fifteen years, we doctors are encountering more and more incidences of growth-plate damage in the shoulders of preadolescent boys.

The growth plates represent the weakest links in the young musculo-skeletal chain. In the adult these areas are no longer present, and stress is absorbed instead by ligaments, tendons, and the bone itself. But in the shoulders of baseball-playing youngsters up to the age of fifteen, it is the growth plate at the top of the humerus that is required to bear much of the stress in repeated hard-throwing or pitching (see Fig. 6).

What occurs is this: with repeated stress on the growth plate at the top of the humerus, the bone loses its blood supply and becomes devitalized. The symptoms are acute pain in the shoulder upon any attempt to throw a ball, followed by an insistent dull ache that becomes more severe with subsequent attempts to throw. Similar ailments can develop in and around the growth plates of the elbow in preadolescent tennis players as well.

Fortunately, damaged or devitalized bone regenerates and heals. However, if youngsters are allowed to continue competing when this situation develops, their shoulders or elbows can develop serious complications and weaknesses that will affect their joint function later in life.

Hence, I caution you to be on the lookout for these signs in your own sports-minded children. If symptoms develop, take them to your physician and have the painful area X-rayed (growth-plate damage about the shoulder or elbow shows up readily on X rays). If the picture reveals incipient bone devitalization, take them off the sport until they reach the age of fifteen at least.

9

YOUR HIP MISERIES

The hip joint is similar to the shoulder joint in many ways. First, it is a ball-and-socket joint. Second, it connects the leg to the torso in much the same way that the shoulder connects the arm. Third, its site is jam-packed with muscles, ligaments, tendons, nerves, and blood vessels. In short, just as the shoulder is the junction box of all the functions of the arm which stem from within the torso, so too is the hip with respect to all the functions of the leg.

The one major difference lies in the fact that the hip is a weight-bearing joint, whereas the shoulder is not. Because of this, the hip is a much more firmly rooted ball-and-socket affair than the shoulder. The result is, of course, that the hip is not capable of the wide range of motion that the shoulder is. But this has its benefits, too, the major one of which is that the hip is not as subject to as many sports-related ailments as the shoulder.

Indeed, serious hip-ailments are thankfully rare as compared to other joint areas of the body. I say thankfully because the hip, being the most massive and complex joint of the body, is the most difficult to deal with from a treatment point of view. Thankfully, also, most sports-related injuries and ailments of the hip do not involve the joint itself but the muscles, tendons, and bursae that surround it. Not that we should be thankful that such ailments exist; but if they have to exist, at least they are where we can readily get at them.

YOUR HIP

Your hip joint is composed of two bones—the pelvis and the femur, or thigh bone. The pelvis, you'll recall from our discussion of the back, is made up of the *sacrum* in the rear, the *two ilia* on the sides, and the two *pubic* bones in front, each with a lower bony projection called the *ischium*.

On the outer fore side of each ilium, where it joins the pubis and ischium, a cup is formed. This is called the *acetabulum* of the hip, and it is the socket-part of the joint. It is angled slightly forward and downward.

At the top of the thigh bone a cylindrical "neck" projects inward, slightly forward and upward at a thirty degree angle. The end of this neck expands in a bulbous fashion. Called the "head" of the femur, it inserts into the acetabulum, or socket, and becomes the "ball" of the joint.

If this was all there was to the hip joint, the hip itself would have an extremely wide range of motion.

But now we come to its ligaments, which, as you know, are those body tissues that primarily hold bones together. The ligaments that tie the outer surfaces of the femur to the pelvis are very strong, and their binding effect on the two bones reduces the hip's range of motion.

Most ordinary sports injuries and ailments affect the outside rather than the inside of the joint. Generally, it is only when severe stresses are applied to the hip, such as in automobile accidents or high falls, that the hip joint itself becomes damaged. The other kind of joint damage, of course, is that which brings about arthritis. I shall discuss this later.

The rest of the joint is composed of the usual synovial membrane, for lubrication and nourishment purposes, and its tough capsule. Overlaying the capsule all around are the numerous muscles that move and further support the hip. Most hip miseries arise in these muscles and in their related tendons and bursae.

The hip has four basic motions—flexion, extension, abduction, and adduction—plus all four in a kind of rotatory combination. The primary muscles that *flex* the hip—that is, allow the thigh to move forward—are the *rectus femoris*, which forms part of the quadriceps muscle-group along the front of the thigh; and the *ilio psoas*, which originates in the lower spine, passes through the pelvis, and attaches to the front and inner portions of the thigh bone just below the neck of the femur. The point of attachment is a bony prominence called the *lesser trochanter*.

The primary muscles that *abduct* the hip, that move the thigh sideways from the midline of the body, originate around the top margins of the pelvis, descend over the hip joint, and attach just below it to another bony prominence, the *greater trochanter*, located be-

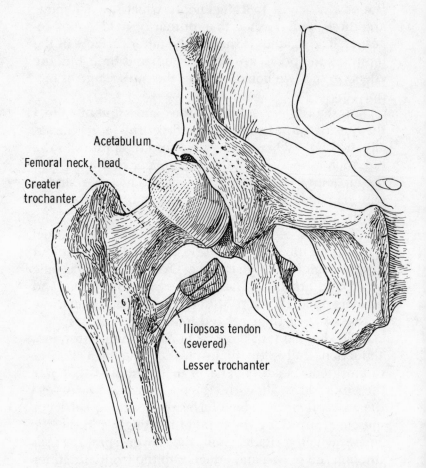

FIG. 16.   *The hip joint; note especially the greater
and lesser trochanter, the sites of most hip miseries.*

low the head of the femur. Remember that all these
muscle attachments are made through tendons, upon
which lie bursae.

The muscles that *adduct* the hip—bring the thigh
in toward the body's midline—originate along the

lower margins of the pelvis and attach to the inner portions of the thigh bone.

The primary muscles that *extend* the hip—permit the thigh to move rearward—are the old familiar *gluteus maximi,* or "glutes," which travel from the back of the pelvis, through the buttocks, to the rear of the thigh bone just below the hip joint.

You can see, then, that the hip is covered thickly with muscles on all sides. This is really all you need to know about your hip to understand the miseries you suffer—if in fact you do suffer them—in your hip region. The only other items of significance are two bursae. One, the *greater trochanteric bursa,* covers the greater trochanter, where the abductor tendon attaches your abductor muscles to the lateral side of your femur. The other is the bursa over the tendon that attaches your iliopsoas muscle—the long muscle that comes down from your back through your pelvis—to the lesser trochanter on the inner side of your femur. Each of these plays a role in the miseries I'm about to describe.

HIP POINTER

"Hip pointer" is a sports term for severe pain and inflammation over the greater trochanter of your femur, just lateral to and slightly forward of the hip joint itself. This pain can come about in two ways—either through a direct blow (this is the "point" of your hip closest to the skin) or through a recurrent strain on the abductor muscles which results in continued stress on the muscles' site of attachment, again at the greater trochanter.

Either way, inflammation and swelling of the bursa

occurs, and the pain can be so intense and disabling that the ailment will also be mistaken for a fractured hip, especially when its precipitating cause is a direct blow.

When the pain and inflammation are the result of a blow, you can expect a two-to-three-week recuperation period. It should be treated immediately with ice, and then allowed to heal itself through time and a moratorium on strenuous activities (often the pain will be so great that you won't feel up to any type of activity, strenuous or otherwise).

When the pain and inflammation seem to develop spontaneously—when they have no apparent precipitating cause—the probability is that you have a tendency to overindulge each time you engage in a "leg" sport that calls for frequent, sudden, and extended hip-abduction. This could be any number of sports—tennis, skiing, horseback riding, and dozens of others. What it means is that by constantly abducting poorly conditioned muscles, you fatigue them. The tired and weakened muscles, unable to stand up under the punishment, transfer their overloads to your thigh bone. Your bone has other things to worry about, however, so it hands the stresses back to the connecting tissue at the greater trochanter. The burden falls upon the tissue, and it becomes inflamed. It, in turn, causes the greater trochanteric bursa to become inflamed and swell.

Since this is a progressive ailment—much like tennis elbow—you will usually not be terribly conscious of it until it is well upon you and regularly interfering with your ability to play your sport. Treatment is much the same as with tennis elbow: rest, followed, if necessary, by a cortisone injection to hasten healing, and then improvement in the tone and strength of your hip's abductor muscles.

BOWLER'S HIP

Bowler's hip refers to pain and inflammation which seem to be centered deep inside the hip. It gets its name because it is so frequently found among bowlers, but it can, in fact, occur quite easily in any sport that includes extensive and recurrent hip extension coupled with twisting motions of the lower back. The basic bowling motion, however, probably best illustrates how it comes about.

Bowler's hip is an inflammation of the *iliopsoas tendon* and its bursae, where they attach the iliopsoas muscle to the lesser trochanter—which is to say, on the inner part of the femur just below the hip joint. The basic bowling motion is a long forward stride in which the leg opposite the bowling arm is suddenly extended, with the hip and knee sharply flexed, as the ball is released. This motion (or anything like it), when performed again and again, tends to fatigue the iliopsoas muscle—especially when it ends with a twisting motion of the back.

As the abductor muscles convey applied stresses to their tendons, the tired and recurrently overstrained iliopsoas passes the stress to its connecting tissues at the femur, and progressive pain and inflammation result.

This is not a serious ailment, but it is annoying for the chronic pain it produces deep in the hip during athletic activities that require such hip extension. Initially, plain rest is the best prescription, followed of course by strengthening, through hip-extension exercises, of the ilio psoas and the other hip-extensor muscles. In stubborn cases, cortisone can help.

GOLFER'S HIP

There are several other aches and pains which are centered in the region of the hip, but these usually have to do with tears and pulls of the muscles. I shall cover them later in the chapter on muscle problems.

It should go without saying that any time you suffer a blow to your hip, and it is accompanied by severe pain and disability, you should immediately see a physician. More likely than not his examination will reveal only a hip pointer or a bruise, but until you and he know for sure, neither of you will rest easy.

This leaves us with one last hip-ailment to discuss —that elusive and deceptively named source of pain and aggravation called "golfer's hip." I say that it is deceptively named because it is a condition that often occurs in people who have never seen a golf course— indeed, in people who are not even athletic. It is, however, common among golfers, which is understandable, because the golf swing is probably the only athletic maneuver in which the hips go through so great a range of various motions in conjunction with the back.

Golfer's hip can certainly develop as a result of playing golf. When it does, it is usually caused by a faulty swing, which leads to abnormal stresses on the hip muscles created by the improper distribution of forces. But golfer's hip is usually nothing more than a preexisting bursitis of the hip that is aggravated when one happens to play golf.

Bursitis of the hip, as I have indicated, usually occurs in one or both of two hip bursae. The first we have already had a look at: it is the greater trochanteric bursa, which is situated at the "point" of the hip, the greater trochanter, and overlies the abductor muscles' attachment.

This bursa tends to become inflamed, you'll recall, as a result of the repeated contraction of the abductor muscles when they are fatigued or weak. Now, the basic stance in golf is the legs-spread, or hips-abducted, stance. The basic motion in the golf swing, aside from the rotation of the shoulders, is the swing and rotation of the hips. When this motion is performed—and especially when it is performed improperly—while the hips are abducted, it tends to put an even greater strain on the abductor muscles than usual.

The average weekend golfer goes around in about ninety strokes, which means that he or she stresses the greater trochanteric bursa of each hip ninety times in a two-to-three hour tour of the course. Add to that figure almost as many, or even twice as many, practice swings, and you have anywhere from two hundred to three hundred bursa aggravations during every three-hour match, or roughly one hundred per hour. This is what I would call recurrent and fatiguing aggravation.

We have also had a look at the second significant bursa of the hip—that over the lesser trochanter where the iliopsoas muscle from the lower back attaches. This is called the *iliopsoas bursa,* and we have seen how it can become inflamed in athletic maneuvers such as are common to bowling.

Another way it can become chronically inflamed is in sudden twisting and rotating motions of the lower back and hip while the legs are straight and the feet firmly planted on the ground. The force of the twist, instead of being dissipated into the ground through a swing of the legs, is concentrated in the ilio psoas muscle's tendinous terminus at the hip. This is because, while the hip and back are swinging in a lateral plane, the legs remain stationary. Again, the stress and overload pile up at the muscles' site of attachment, and inflammation of the bursae—one on either hip—follows.

These inflammations, either singly or in combination, are what we know as golfer's hip. When they develop as a result of playing golf, they are caused by the constant and recurring traumas produced by a faulty swing. When they already exist for other reasons, playing golf will merely aggravate them.

The treatment of golfer's hip is similar to the treatment of other hip ailments, for, as we now know, the most common sports-associated miseries of the hip are nothing more than forms of bursitis. Two helpful adjuncts to the permanent relief of golfer's hip would be, of course, strengthening the abductor and iliopsoas muscles through exercises, and developing a proper golf swing.

TWO SIMPLE EXERCISES

Exercise 1. Hip Abductor Side-Raise
Lie on your side with your legs extended, the upper leg resting on the lower one. Slowly raise the upper leg, keeping it straightened, as high as it will go. Hold for a count of ten, then return *slowly* to the starting position. Do twenty repetitions, then change to your other side and repeat the exercise with your other leg. When you can do twenty repetitions easily on both sides, add ankle weights in progressive two-pound increments.

Exercise 2. Sprinter's Stretch
Assume modified sprinter's position with one leg thrust straight out behind you, foot braced against a

wall, your other leg tucked up under your chest, and your hands planted solidly on the floor in front of you. Let your body drop toward the floor on the straight-leg side, then raise it up again, using only your hip muscles for power. Repeat ten times, then reverse legs and do ten times again. This exercise stretches the flexor muscles of your hip.

Exercise 3.   Leg Swing.

Sit on the edge of a table or desk. Let your leg hang free over the forward edge from the knee. Press both hands, one on top of the other, against the middle portion of the thigh. Then attempt to lift the thigh off the table while resisting with your hands. Hold for a count of five, then relax. Start with 10 repetitions and work up to 30.

10

YOUR WRIST AND HAND MISERIES

No structures of our body are more important to us than our hands. Our hands enable us to cope with our environment, to bring things into our reach, and to accomplish whatever our minds set out for us to do. Indeed, not only our brains set us apart from the rest of the animal world, but also the ability of our thumbs and fingers to function in opposition.

Our hands, however, are nothing without our wrists. Our wrists are the "puppet strings" of our hands, and unless we can maintain their structural integrity, our hands will not be able to do all we require of them in our different athletic endeavors. So in this chapter we shall consider the wrist and hand together.

The knowledge you have gained so far about the other joints of your body should give you a head start in understanding the nature of your wrists and the various parts of your hands. The wrist is composed of many small joints. The many joints of the fingers are mini hinge joints, not unlike the knee in their basic design. What enables these joints to move is a marvelous collection of muscles, tendons, and ligaments which also serve to support them.

From the viewpoint of anatomy, the hand begins at the wrist. The wrist is the junction of the two forearm bones, the radius and ulna, and four *carpal* bones that form the hand's upper segment. These bones, which are set in a row across the width of the upper hand, are blocklike and articulate with the cartilage-lubricated ends of the radius and ulna.

Set in a similiar row below these four bones is a second row of blocklike carpals. These bones articulate above with the carpals of the first row and below with the bases of the thumb-and-finger bones, the *metacarpals,* to give the wrist and hand their suppleness and mobility.

All these joints are held together by a network of ligaments and synovial capsules which provide lubrication, nourishment, and further support.

In addition to the major wrist joint there is another joint at the site which is also important. This is the *radioulnar joint.* It is situated between the ends of the two forearm bones, and enables them to articulate with one another, or slide against one another, during various motions of the wrist joint and forearm. Situated in this joint is a small meniscus, or cartilage, as in the knee, which eases the articulation of the joint. Damage to this cartilage through recurrent overstresses on the wrist in pronation or supination can cause a chronic and painful stiffening-disability in the wrist.

The metacarpal bones are the long bones whose heads form the large knuckles of our hand and whose bases articulate with the adjoining carpal bones of the wrist. From the knuckles of the metacarpals, and articulating with them, extend the *phalanges,* or the bones of the fingers.

All the fingers, except for the thumb, have three phalanges. The *proximal phalanges* are the bones that go from the knuckles to the first joints of the fingers. The *middle phalanges* go from the first joints to the second. And the *distal phalanges* go from the second joints to the fingertips.

The thumb has only two phalanges—the *proximal,* which runs from the knuckles of the thumb to its joint, and the *distal,* which runs from the joint to the tip.

The knuckle joints of the fingers and thumb, called the *metacarpal-phalangeal joints,* are basically saddle joints—they are capable of both flexion-extension and a certain amount of lateral and rotatory motion as well, especially at the thumb. The nine joints further up the fingers and thumb, called the *interphalangeal joints,* are strictly hinge joints, and are capable of only straight-line flexion and extension.

As with the much larger knee joint, the interphalangeal joints of the fingers are held together and braced on each side primarily by small *collateral ligaments.* These are the checkreins that prevent the joints from moving from side to side. They are also the structures that become damaged when a finger is dislocated or "jammed."

The most important structures in the hand, however, are the long tendons from the forearms. There are certain intrinsic muscles in the hand itself—muscles which originate in the palm and insert into the fingers

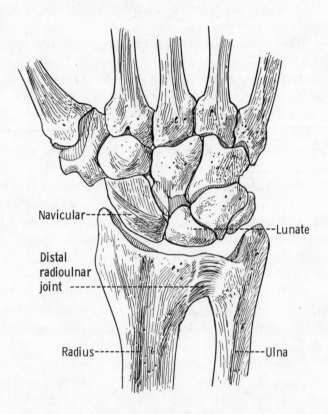

FIG. 17. *A skeletal view of your wrist joint and hand, from above. Note the radioulnar joint, held together by a ligament, and the navicular bone.*

—but the hand and fingers get most of their motor power from the muscles of the forearm. This power is transferred through the wrist by means of a complex network of tendons which, as they attach to the various bones of the hand and fingers, provide their joints with the ability to flex or extend.

You will recall from my chapter on the elbow how the forearm extensor and flexor muscles work on that joint. These muscles also extend and flex the wrist. Beyond the wrist—that is, in the hand— they extend and flex the fingers through a series of long tendons that attach to the metacarpals and phalanges. It is precisely this continuation of the forearm muscles into the hand that accounts for the fact that a handshake, or some other form of gripping or squeezing, causes intense pain in an inflamed elbow.

Remember that a muscle must attach to the far side of a joint to move it. The flexor and extensor tendons, which are, in effect, continuations of the forearm flexor and extensor muscles, extend in branches through the hand and all the way to the distal phalanges of the fingers and thumb, attaching to the phalanges beyond each of the interphalangeal joints. The flexor tendons attach on the undersides of the bones, while the extensor tendons attach on the top sides. All these tendons, of course, work together.

Most of the muscles in the hand itself are there to aid in the flexion and extension of the fingers and thumb, and in spreading the fingers apart and bringing them together. In addition to these muscles, the thumb has a special muscle at its base called the *opponens* muscle. Its function is, as you have undoubtedly guessed, to provide the thumb with its rotatory capability.

All these muscles are attached to the finger bones through their own tendons. As you can gather, then, most miseries of the hands and wrists, excepting fractures and arthritis, involve the musculo-tendinous tissue of these regions, particularly around the many joints that exist there.

SWINGER'S WRIST

No, swinger's wrist does not refer to an occupational hazard of the modern, organized practice of "sexual swinging," or mate-swapping. It does refer to many other forms of athletic activity, though, particularly to those in which one holds a racket, bat, or club in one's hands and strikes a ball with it. As an athletic ailment, it occurs most frequently among tennis players, but is also a common hazard of golfing.

Swinger's wrist arises for pretty much the same reasons that tennis elbow comes about, although it is a markedly different kind of disorder: overload at the wrist at the moment of force or impact, due to a faulty swing, is the chief cause, aided of course by under-developed forearm muscles.

Swinger's wrist, to describe it medically, is an alteration of the normal articulation, and an inflammation of the radio-ulnar joint—not the main wrist joint, but that joint between the two forearm bones at the wrist which enables them to move against one another during various motions of the wrist itself. The condition is caused, in tennis, by hitting the ball with the wrist in an "ulnar-deviated" position—in other words, with a faulty backhand stroke, the same stroke that also brings about tennis elbow.

It is almost certain that when a tennis player consistently and repeatedly hits a backhand when the ball is far in front of the body, the weight is on the forward foot, and the elbow is high and bent, he or she will develop tennis elbow. What usually follows is that the enthusiast will continue to play and, without correcting his or her swing, but now favoring the elbow, will begin to hit the same shot so that most of the force and excess stress is transferred to the wrist.

Since the stroke is habitually faulty, before the onset of tennis elbow its power would come from the forearm-elbow region of the arm. *After* the onset of tennis elbow and its attendant pain, the improper stroke's power must be generated in the forearm-wrist region. This means that there must be an excessive snapping of the wrist at impact, with the radio-ulnar joint already in an extreme state of stress due to the faulty position of the arm in the elbow-up position.

Repeated shocks are driven into the overstressed joint, tearing fibers in its meniscus, or cartilage, and causing inflammation around its attachments to the bone. This is, for the most part, an affliction of the inexperienced or recreational player, but I have also seen it in top-notch tournament competitors who hit the two-handed backhand with extreme wrist roll. It also occurs frequently in the wrists of golfers who have a tendency to let their clubheads hit the ground before they hit the ball.

In mild cases of radio-ulnar joint inflammation, treatment follows the usual rest-and-rehabilitation routine, with the possible administration of cortisone to hasten the reduction of the inflammation. In severe cases, surgery may be required to excise the cartilage and restore painless wrist function. Of course, treatment will be of little help in the future prevention of this condition unless steps are taken to learn the proper swings and strokes.

BASEBALL FINGER

How many of us have gone to catch a ball—whether it be a baseball, football, basketball, or vol-

leyball—and suddenly found one of our fingers painfully jammed? Known as baseball finger because it occurs most frequently in that sport, "jammed finger" is
an affliction common to many different athletic activities, and although it is properly speaking an injury, if
not treated correctly it can have chronic complications
which, by preventing proper gripping, can interfere
with your enjoyment of many recreational sports.

Baseball finger occurs when a hard, moving object
impacts against the tip of an inadvertently extended
finger and forces its distal and/or middle interphalangeal hinge joints to suddenly hyperflex backward or
bend to the side. Either way, there is a stretch and,
depending on the force, possibly a tear of the collateral
ligaments of the joints, causing swelling, inmobility,
and intense pain.

Immediate treatment consists of placing ice on the
area to keep swelling down, determining through X
rays that no fractures exist, and immobilizing the finger
for a short period. It is wrong, under all circumstances,
to immobilize the finger by putting it in a splint for any
length of time. The best way to immobilize it is to tape
it to its next adjoining finger so that limited joint articulation can occur without undue bending of the injured
interphalangeal joints.

Unless the collateral ligaments are totally torn
(which is unusual), no further measures above and
beyond the normal healing process will be necessary.
Depending on the extent of the tear, most baseball
fingers will return to normal joint function, although
with more extensive tears there will be slight instability
at the affected joint. This instability will not be enough
to interfere with one's normal manual activities, but

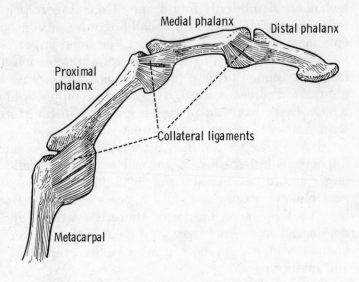

FIG. 18.   *The bones of the finger, their three joints, and the ligaments of one side.*

may make the finger more vulnerable to further "jam-mings" when even lighter forces are applied to it.

MALLET FINGER

Mallet finger is a more serious version of baseball finger, with more potentially disabling consequences. It occurs when the tip of the finger is impacted by a moving object such as a ball, and the distal or farthest inter-phalangeal joint is hyperflexed (bent) at the same time as its extensor tendon is contracting. In other words, as one is opening or extending one's finger it is struck on the tip, and its distal joint is forcibly bent downward.

What happens then is basically the collision of two opposing forces within the finger: the flexing force vs. the extending force. Something's got to give. And since the flexing force of the impacting object is greater than the extending force of the joint's extensor tendon, the tendon gives.

Actually, that is imprecise. The tendons in the finger are extremely tough and resistant to tearing, and the distal extensor tendons are no exception. So it is not the tendon itself that gives; rather, it struggles to combat the overload brought about by the impact. The result is that the tendon pulls a piece of bone off the spot at which it attaches to the distal phalanx. In other words, the extensor tendon is no longer attached, or is only partially attached, to the bone beyond the joint. It is therefore no longer, or only marginally, able to extend the joint. Hence the joint remains in a flexed position and the finger takes on a mallet-head configuration.

This deformity may become permanent unless it is treated immediately and properly. Early treatment is simple: it calls for putting the finger in a splint, with its distal end in extension until the tendon-bone attachment can heal back together again through natural bone-and-tendon tissue regeneration. If this treatment is not undertaken immediately, however, and the deformity is permitted to become permanent, its correction can only be achieved surgically.

BOWLER'S THUMB

Although the incidence of other hand ailments spreads across the whole spectrum of sports activities, here is a misery that is limited almost exclusively to bowlers. The reasons should be obvious.

In bowling, the bowler grips a quite heavy ball between his or her thumb and first two fingers, all of which are inserted into holes made for that purpose. Most bowlers like to put a little "English" on the ball as they release it; indeed, this is necessary in order for the ball to strike the pins at a desirable angle rather than straight on.

Putting English on the ball means an inward twist or pronation of the wrist as the ball is released. Hold your hand in front of you, with your thumb and first two fingers extended, and abruptly pronate your wrist. You will notice that the upper part of your thumb automatically tucks under and flexes in toward your palm as you reach full pronation.

In bowling, because your thumb is imprisoned in the ball's thumbhole until release, this natural thumb flexion is prevented. As you release the ball your two fingers have already begun to slip out of their holes, but your thumb stays in its hole until the last possible moment so as to maintain control over the ball's spin. When it finally releases, your wrist is in extreme pronation. Free of the thumbhole, your thumb, which has been straining to remain in extension while in the hole, suddenly and belatedly flexes in toward your palm. This flexion occurs later than it would if you were pronating your wrist without gripping the ball.

The repeated abduction and extension strain, followed by the sudden adduction and flexion of your thumb, tends to fatigue the muscles around it which aid in these motions. This fatigue is transferred to the connecting tendons, especially to those of the *opponens* muscle at the thumb's base, and inflammation—often becoming chronic—follows.

Treatment is as usual for such tendon-bone irritations. But prevention is simpler. The two most sensible ways to prevent it are: (a) exercise your thumb muscles, particularly by squeezing a small ball between your thumb and first two fingers; and (b) reduce the spin you try to put on the ball.

NAVICULAR FRACTURES

The navicular bone of the wrist is the outermost of the four blocklike carpal bones that are arrayed in a row across the base of your hand. It is the bone that faces the end of the forearm's radius on the wrist's outer side and articulates with it to form the outer part of the wrist joint.

Now, I'm not trying to make a doctor out of you. That is why I haven't dealt to any great extent in this book with serious athletic injuries, fractures, and dislocations. However, it is important that you understand what a navicular fracture is. It is very common among recreational athletes, and when it is overlooked or ignored—as it often is since it's not extremely painful—it can create permanent wrist debility.

Whether you are a tennis player or a skier, a volleyball enthusiast or a touch-football fiend, there are going to be times when you will fall. Whenever we fall forward, our natural instinct is to stick out our hands to break the fall and protect our bodies. Often we are successful in this objective, but sometimes our success creates further problems. We land full-force on the heels of our hands just below our thumbs, sending tremendous shock stresses up the navicular and radial aspects of our wrists. Frequently, a fracture will occur as a result in one or both of these bones.

When it does, there will be pain and discomfort, but sometimes not much more than when we simply sprain a wrist. So we will tend to ignore it, or at least allow it to rest in the hopes that the pain and swelling will go away by themselves.

This is a mistake because navicular fractures can be disastrous, and unwittingly ignoring them can result in a permanent wrist disability. Thus, any time you fall on your wrist and suffer what seems to be more than minor pain over the outer aspect of the joint, you should consult a physician so that he can confirm or rule out the existence of a navicular fracture.

Why is this so important? Simply because a navicular fracture in many cases will sever the blood supply to the bone, or at least to half of it. With the blood supply severed, the bone will not regenerate, the fracture will not unite again, and the blood-deprived portion of the bone will die. And with the bone, or part of it, dead, the wrist will become painfully disabling, requiring reconstructive surgery.

11

YOUR FOOT MISERIES

We've already had a brief look at part of the foot in our chapter on ankle ailments. We've discussed the ankle bone itself—the *talus*—and the *calcaneum,* or heel bone, on which the talus sits.

The foot, of course, is the anatomical equivalent in the lower extremities of the hand. Thus, the talus and calcaneum are similar to the first row of carpal bones at the base of the hand. In anatomy, they are called the *large tarsal* bones of the foot.

Forward of the ankle and heel bones is a collection of five smaller blocklike bones which form the arch of the foot and are called the *small tarsal* bones. Of these, the bone on the inner upper side of the arch—also called *navicular*—articulates with the ankle bone. A larger bone on the outer lower side of the arch, the *cuboid,* articulates with the heel bone.

The other three small tarsal bones, known as *cunei-form* bones, along with the forward margin of the cuboid, connect with five long bones that run to the base of the toes. These five bones are the *metatarsals,* and are akin to the metacarpals of the hand. They in turn connect with the bones of the toes, of which there are two *phalanges* in the large toe (equivalent to the thumb) and three in the other four toes (equivalent to the fingers). Of course each of the toes' phalanges have between them interphalangeal joints, just as do the fingers.

The usual complement of muscles, tendons, ligaments, and joint capsules exists in the foot to complete its musculo-skeletal construction. The only remarkable thing about this construction, as compared to other regions of the body, is in the arch of the foot. The rest of the foot, along with its common ailments, is, if you'll forgive the pun, pretty pedestrian.

There are actually two distinct arches in the foot. The first and most noticeable one is the *longitudinal arch,* the arch along the inner top margin of the foot. The second is the *metatarsal arch,* which lies across the foot beneath the heads of the long metatarsal bones. The ancient Greeks discovered that an arch will support and distribute weight much more effectively than a flat surface; thus they began building arches in all their temples. This was a case of art imitating nature, for nature had long previously determined that the arch of the human foot was the best means of supporting and distributing the weight of the human body.

FALLEN ARCHES

The arch of the foot is held in suspension by ligament and muscle. But not all arches maintain their
structural integrity. Some people are born with "fallen
arches," or flat feet. Others develop this condition due
to inherent weaknesses in their foot-ligaments and
muscles. In either case, many athletic activities can
turn into painful, fatiguing, and frustrating pursuits.*

Many of us can recall that certain flat-feet conditions were one of the primary forms of disqualification
for the military draft during World War II and
thereafter. The theory was that sufferers of flat feet
could not march and were therefore useless. Indeed, in
years past many a parent brought an otherwise healthy
teenage son to me in order to persuade me to declare
him, when he was due to report for his draft physical,
a victim of flat feet. More than one anxious parent went
home sorely disappointed to discover that his or her
offspring had perfectly normal feet.

But the military's rationale, back before the days of
the nonmarching army, was correct. Rigid, flat feet
created more problems for the services than they
solved. And until recently, they created more problems
for the recreational athlete than they solved. Today,
however, with the advances that have been made in
shoe construction and artificial arch supports, the pain
and fatigue of flat feet should no longer be a problem
to the athletically inclined.

If you have flat feet and haven't already done so,
you can easily take the necessary measures to correct

---

*Of course, not all flat feet are painful. Many great athletes have flat feet.
In children, feet appear flat until about two years of age.

them by employing a variety of orthopedic devices doctors can prescribe. The best way to achieve this is through foot supports specially molded to your feet and designed according to a physician's diagnosis and order. But first you should *visit* a knowledgeable physician so that he can determine the nature and extent of your condition and advise you in the *proper* approach to alleviating it. Fallen arches cannot be restored to normal, they can only be compensated for. I have seen many patients who diagnose themselves as having flat feet and then go out on their own and purchase the completely *wrong* kind of shoe or device for their condition. By so doing, they exacerbate their problem and end up with such foot maladies as bunions, hammer toes, and painful calluses and corns.

Those who are born and grow up with flat feet don't have it as bad as those whose arches fall later on in life. In the former, the longitudinal arch fails to elevate, but as the foot grows its bones, muscles, and ligaments adjust so that there are no excessively painful stresses during normal activities. They do tend to walk on the inner margins of their feet, however, which causes a permanent inversion of the ankles and potential weaknesses there.

In people who develop fallen arches later in life, the problem is not so simple, especially when it is the metatarsal arch that falls.

CLAW TOES AND HAMMER TOES

The metatarsal arch is formed by the heads, or rounded ends, of all five metatarsal bones. The arch they form supports the forefoot and allows body weight to be transferred from the lateral, or outer, border of the foot to the big toe in a smooth, even fashion. Muscle balance around the toes—that is, the synergy between the flexor and extensor muscles of the toes—maintains this orderly transfer of weight and power so that it is effortless and painless. However, when inbalance occurs—when some muscles are stronger than others and overpull the toes in one direction—contracture and deformity of the toes occur. Two common types of deformity are *claw toes* and *hammer toes.*

Claw toes is the condition that arises when the toes are hyperextended at their base joints (the metacarpalphalangeal joints) and hyperflexed at their interphalangeal joints. This condition occurs in conjunction with a depressed or "fallen" metatarsal arch of the foot. The effect of the clawing thrusts the bottoms of the metatarsal heads into prominence on the underside of the foot, creating bony knobs under which painful calluses are formed. Special metatarsal pads and "toe-slings" help to relieve the discomfort of the condition, but often the orthopedic surgeon needs to resort to surgical procedures in order to produce long-lasting relief.

A true hammer-toe condition is somewhat different than claw toes. Hammer toes may be congenital, or else may develop as a result of faulty foot-posture and muscle imbalance. The base joints of the toes are generally straight, but the first interphalangeal joint is fixed in an almost ninety-degree flexion so that the tips of the toes are pressed against the ground. In this case, painful calluses develop under the tips of the toes. Although special pads can be used to alleviate the discomfort, hammer toes are best treated through surgery for permanent relief. The procedure is simple and reliable in the hands of an orthopedic surgeon and consists of resectioning the hyperflexed toe joints and fusing them straight.

BUNIONS

Not all hammer-toe conditions are produced by fallen metatarsal arches, but many do develop therefrom. Nor do all bunion ailments come from fallen arches, although, again, many are their direct result. Except among people who actually suffer from bunions, I find a great deal of confusion over the question of exactly what they are. For some reason their name tends to provoke laughter whenever a television comedian cracks a joke about them, but to those of you who suffer from them they are no laughing matter.

What are bunions? Their name, however humorous, should give you a clue. Bunions have to do with bone. More specifically, they are abnormal enlargements of bone. And more specifically still, they are abnormal enlargements in the heads of the metatarsal bones—where they meet the phalanges of the toes.

A bunion is actually an abnormality at the metatarsal head. It usually occurs at the big toe, but may also develop in the little toe, as well. Through constant strain at these sites—due to either fallen-arch pressures or to tight shoes—the head of the metatarsal bones become enlarged.

In the joint of the big toe, this enlargement eventually produces a bone spur that grows over the inner aspect of the metatarsal head. Simultaneously the toe itself deviates outward, often pushing the adjoining toe upward. A bursa is formed around the bony spur, and if excessive pressure from tight shoes is applied, it becomes inflamed, swollen, and very painful. The bunion of the little toe—often called a "bunionette"—comes about in a similar manner.

When they become severe, bunions can be removed surgically. In milder cases rest and cortisone can help. But prevention should be the primary goal, and this can be achieved by relieving the pressures on the affected sites through the use of appropriately designed shoes and arch supports. Proper shoe wear is the best advice that I can give anyone who has bunions or who does not want to develop them.

CORNS

Another kind of growth in the foot are skin growths. Corns are outgrowths of thick tissue which occur on the top of the toes as a reaction to pressure. We often see them in people with various degrees of claw toes, and they develop as a result of constant shoe-rubbing over the flexed and raised interphalangeal joints. And, of course, they are a regular feature in women who wear tight, narrow-toed shoes.

Corns are not serious, but they are painful and *can* produce serious complications. People with corns tend to favor the forward areas of their feet when walking or running. This produces abnormal stresses on the other structures of the feet, and any number of breakdowns can occur as a result. The best way to defeat corns, of course, is to wear more sensible and loose-fitting shoes, but I know from experience that such counsel is destined to go unheeded. We might say that corns are more of a psychological ailment than a physical one and demand psychological treatment—that is, for people to stop wearing shoes that are too small and too pinched, they must be psychologically convinced that their feet are *not* too big, and persuaded to embark on sensible daily shoe habits.

TENNIS TOE

Tennis toe is rapidly catching up with tennis elbow as the most prevalent court ailment, according to Dr. Richard Gibbs, a New York dermatologist. The disorder occurs when a player repeatedly stops short—say, after dashing to the net—and jams his or her large toe against the front of the sneaker. Contributing factors are the new, narrow, hard-toed European tennis shoes that have lately become fashionable, and their improved-traction soles.

In the old days we used to play with soft-toed sneakers that would slide around a good deal on the court's surface. Even when we stopped short and our toes rammed into the front of the sneaker, the force would cause the sole of the sneaker to slide a bit forward, providing a certain amount of built-in "give" and dissipating the pressures on our toes. With the new style sneakers—the ones with the hard, narrow toes and nonslip soles—such "give" does not occur.

When the modern tennis player jams a big toe into the front of his or her new-style sneaker, the result is the rupture of small blood vessels beneath the toenail, which produces discoloration, swelling, and pain. Indeed, when enough vessels are ruptured the nail will lose its blood supply, die, and fall off, making further activities quite uncomfortable until the nail has had a chance to grow back.

Tennis toe should be self-treated immediately by the application of cold compresses, and should be given enough rest-time to recover. Again, of course, common sense dictates that in order to prevent its recurrence you should consign your new European shoes to the bonfire and return to the old-fashioned slip-and-slide kind. I have no desire to deprive the European manufacturers of their right to sell their tennis shoes on our shores, but I do think you are well-advised to exercise *your* right not to buy them—no matter how fashionable the advertisements make them appear.

There are, as you undoubtedly know, a variety of other foot ailments I could discuss—for instance, athlete's foot, calluses, blisters—but they all involve the same concept I have been emphasizing throughout this chapter: the use of proper footwear.

Proper footwear in your athletic endeavors can go a long way to eliminating most foot miseries. It almost seems to go without saying, but I'll say it anyway: if you always make sure you have clean and well-fitting shoes or boots, your feet will remain free of many superficial, chronic ailments that might otherwise plague you. One of our most enduring myths has been the one which claims that to be good athletes we must wear tight-fitting shoes, boots, or sneakers—on the theory that they give our feet the best support. History has exploded this myth, and all that remains is for you to accept history's judgment. In sports, our feet are our most valuable commodities—more important, even, than the kind of skis we choose, the kind of racket we buy, the kind of clubs we tote. Yet most people will invest sixty dollars in a tennis racket, only to follow up by acquiring a cheap pair of sneakers. The same holds true for people in other sports. They put a premium on the tools of their game and ignore those items—their feet—without which the tools are useless.

So—whenever you prepare to start with any sport, start with your most important items of equipment: the things you put on your feet. If your feet are healthy, properly fitted footwear will keep them that way. And if they are in some way abnormal, the same kind of footwear, with appropriate adaptations, will keep the abnormality to a minimum. Who knows, it might even improve it.

12

YOUR MUSCLE MISERIES

I've probably talked about your muscles more frequently than about any other component of your body in the foregoing pages, but always in relation to their supporting and motive roles in the function of your joints. Now the time has come to consider your muscles separately—especially those which are the most common sources of athletic miseries.

Of muscle miseries, there are four major abnormalities—chronic or otherwise—that concern us here. The first is *muscle inflammation*, which I've already covered indirectly during my discussion of various muscle-attachment or tendon miseries such as tennis elbow.

The second is *strained or "pulled" muscle*, probably the most frequent kind of muscle ailment.

The third is *charley horse,* the muscle misery that comes about as a result of a direct blow.

And the fourth is *cramps,* which, when they become chronic, are probably the mildest but most vexing muscle misery of all.

CRAMPS

Again, in my many years of medical practice I have learned that there is a great deal of confusion on the part of the lay public as to the differences between these four types of muscle disorders, and that it is usually the lack of knowledge about the composition and capabilities of the muscles themselves that brings about the high incidence of muscle miseries among recreational or weekend athletes. Hence, before I go on to explain the differences between the four types of muscle disorder and to discuss the principal muscle ailments, a little information on the physiology of muscle is in order—particularly with regard to understanding what muscle cramps are and how they arise.

By now you should be able to clearly visualize your body as a system of bones, muscles, connective tissues, blood vessels, and nerves, with the muscles as the dominant component insofar as your body's bulk is concerned.

The muscle of your body extends outward in layers from the bones of your frame to just beneath your skin. It is composed of pliant, fibrous tissue through which tiny blood vessels—capillaries—and nerve endings flow. The capillaries are there to feed the muscle, that is, supply it with oxygen and nutrients; the nerves are there to innervate it, that is, enable it to contract and relax in response to voluntary or involuntary impulses from the brain.

As muscle is being used it expends energy. In other words, every time a muscle contracts, its fibers require energy to sustain the contraction, and it is constantly using up energy. The necessary energy is provided by the fresh oxygen and sugar fed into the muscle by the blood vessels. As the oxygen is used in the muscle tissues, it manufactures a by-product that accumulates in these tissues. This by-product is called *lactic acid*. Under normal conditions, part of the lactic acid is carried off as waste while new oxygen is being supplied, so that the two substances exist in a kind of natural balance in the muscle tissues.

But when the muscle is overused, an excessive amount of lactic acid is produced due to insufficient oxygen supply. The muscle enters into a condition known as "oxygen debt."

It is when your muscles go into oxygen debt that cramps occur. Cramps are basically nothing more than a form of muscle spasm; that is, as a muscle, or group of muscles, becomes starved for oxygen, it reacts by going into uncontrollable spasm. When the oxygen debt reaches a certain intolerable level, the nerves become alerted and send panic sensory-messages to the brain. Back come equally panicky motor-messages, and the muscles themselves go into panic. The situation is not unlike that of someone choking on a bone; as he gasps for air, he will go into the wildest gyrations imaginable.

There are basically two kinds of cramps of interest to the weekend athlete: *runner's cramps* and *swimmer's cramps.*

RUNNER'S CRAMPS

Runner's cramps are those familiar muscle cramps that occur in the lower leg and foot. They are common in any sport that involves a lot of running and are brought about by two causes—a *precipitating cause* and an *underlying cause*.

The precipitating cause is the fatigue and overloads experienced by the calf and foot muscles during extended running. The underlying cause is due to the fact that our lower extremities naturally receive the least amount of fresh oxygen from our hearts. This is well illustrated by the fact that nonathletic people with poor blood circulation caused by a circulatory disorder often suffer from leg and foot cramps when they are doing nothing more than lying in bed or sitting at their desks.

It all has to do with conditioning. Nonathletic individuals with poor circulation do not get enough oxygen in the muscles of their lower extremities. As lactic acid accumulates in the inactive muscle tissues, even less oxygen becomes available. Suddenly, and for no apparent reason, the muscles go into spasm and cramps ensue.

In the athletic person with poor circulation, or in the person who is a heavy smoker, cramps will occur just as readily during an athletic activity. Here, however, they are additionally provoked by stress on the muscles. They occur least frequently in people who have good peripheral circulation and who don't smoke (you'll recall that smoking inhibits the lungs' capacity to provide proper amounts of fresh oxygen to the blood-supply system).

Thus, chronic muscle cramps of the calf and foot are not just an annoyance, they are a sign that should be heeded. If you are a victim of such cramps during nonathletic activities, you should have your circulation checked. If you are a victim and are a heavy smoker, you should serously think about cutting down or quitting, because it is a sign that your lungs are no longer capable of providing sufficient oxygen to feed your most distant muscles properly. And if you are a weekend athlete and suffer such cramps regularly, you should also have your circulatory system checked.

Cramps come about, as I have said, because your calf and foot muscles have gone into oxygen debt.* When you experience a cramp, you know that the affected muscle is overloaded with lactic acid and is starving for oxygen. The best way to relieve the cramps is to get off your feet and vigorously massage the muscle. Massage stimulates circulation, which in turn increases the delivery of oxygen to the muscle. This enables you to pay off the muscle's oxygen debt much more quickly than if you simply wait for the cramp to subside on its own.

But this is only first aid. Remember, if you are a chronic leg-and-foot cramp sufferer, you should get yourself to a physician so that you can discover and correct the underlying cause.

SWIMMER'S CRAMPS

As children, we were all admonished by our parents never to go in the water for at least an hour after

---

*Cramps also occur in the healthy athlete during very hot weather. These are caused by dehydration—that is, when excessive amounts of body salts and other minerals are lost through perspiration and are not immediately replaced. To avoid "heat cramps," the weekend athlete should swallow salt tablets before and during his or her play.

eating lunch. Of course, being the rebellious creatures we were, many of us ignored these warnings. We lived to tell the tale, and as we grew older we came to believe that the admonition was just another of those myths parents pass along to their children. Then we had children of our own, and, to our surprise, we found ourselves repeating the same stern warning to them. When we do so, most of us don't even think about, or know, the reason for it. All we know is what we were told—swimming after eating is bad for us; it causes cramps and can bring about our premature demise through drowning.

Is it an old wives' tale or isn't it? The answer, I'm afraid is that it's not. Anyone who *has* been attacked by cramps while swimming is the best witness to the validity of the warning. The mechanics of swimmer's cramps follows a scenario similar to that of leg-and-foot cramps in the runner, with oxygen debt playing the leading role. It is only that some of the muscles involved are different.

After we ingest food, our involuntary stomach and intestinal muscles get busy processing it through our gastrointestinal system. We have no conscious control over these muscles, yet while digesting and breaking down the food in our stomach they work with the intensity of a battalion of beavers building a dam. To lend them support, our blood-supply system diverts oxygen from other parts of our body to our gastrointestinal tract.

This is why we so often become sleepy after eating a big meal. Our gastrointestinal muscles are working at a furious rate, draining oxygen from the more distant extremities of our body—our brain, for instance, as well as our legs and arms. It is also why a brisk walk after

eating is helpful to digestion. Copious lungfuls of fresh
air while walking increase our oxygen supply. The oxygen required by our digestive muscles is available in
greater quantities, and there is still enough left over to
feed the rest of our body tissues sufficiently.

But if we venture into the waters of a pool, lake, or
ocean shortly after eating, we find a different situation.
With our involuntary stomach-muscles working over-
time, oxygen debt in our legs, as well as in our stomach
muscles, builds up. When we swim we do not breathe
normally; rather, we take our breaths at longer intervals. This reduces our intake of oxygen, further adding
to the debt.

The body will demand payment either in the stomach first, or in the legs. And when payment is unforth-
coming, the muscles of the stomach or legs, whichever
is suffering the greater oxygen starvation, will respond
with cramps.

Stomach cramps will bend you in half with pain—
you will feel as though you've been hit with the blunt
end of a ramrod. Leg cramps, usually in the calf, will
lock your leg with equal pain. In either case, you will
become helpless in the water, and if you have a panicky
nature you are liable to drown.

The only way to beat this situation, if you are un-
wise enough to swim in deep water after eating, is to
overcome your panic with knowledge. Thrashing
around hysterically in the water will only increase the
cramps and decrease the possibility of your survival.

Shout for help once or twice, but don't spend all
your time shouting. This just uses up more oxygen. Instead, if you can, use your common sense and your
knowledge. You now know that your cramps are caused
by an oxygen debt in the affected muscles, brought

about by a temporary insufficiency of oxygen in your blood stream. Your task, then, is to get more oxygen into your system. How? By taking deep breaths of fresh air.

Tread water as best you can with your arms, keeping the rest of your body still. Overcome your preoccupation with the cramps. Get your mouth clear of the water and take quick, deep breaths of fresh air. If you are able to do this for a minute or so, the likelihood is great that your cramps will abate.

If you spend all your time shouting for help you will just go deeper into oxygen debt and will probably no longer be there by the time rescuers reach you. If you are any distance from potential rescuers, you are better off trying to save yourself by means of the deep-breathing method. Once your cramps have abated, continue the deep breathing for another few minutes so that your body can build up an oxygen surplus. Then either shout for help or slowly make your way in toward shore.

MUSCLE PULLS

Other muscle miseries usually take the form of pulls or tears, although there are also such things as contusions (bruises) and inflammations. Much confusion exists over the differences between a pulled, or torn, muscle and a contused muscle, and between these two and an inflamed muscle. Actually, the differences are simple and can be clearly determined in terms of their respective causes.

A *pulled, or torn, muscle* is caused by the stretching of a muscle beyond its normal conditioned elasticity; fibers in the belly of the muscle tear or pull apart and cause the muscle itself to become painful.

A *contused, or bruised, muscle* is caused by a direct traumatic blow. The tiny blood vessels at the site of the blow burst and hemorrhage, causing the muscle to fill with blood and causing localized pain to develop. The term "charley horse" refers to a contused or bruised muscle. I have no idea where the name comes from; I can only surmise that someone once was kicked by a horse called "Charley" and so-christened the resulting contusion. This injury usually occurs in the thigh.

An *inflamed muscle,* aside from the inflammation caused by tears and bruises, refers less to the muscle itself and more to its tendinous bone-attachment—as in tennis elbow. Although the inflammation is centered in the tendon, usually because of chronic stretching stresses, it can also extend into the muscle itself.

In discussing the most common of these muscle miseries, let's work from the feet up.

PLANTARIS RUPTURE

You've learned that the major muscle in the back of the calf is the *gastrocnemius,* which travels from the Achilles tendon to the back of the femur and aids in the flexing of the knee joint. Buried beneath this massive muscle is a long, thin muscle called the *plantaris,* which is joined at the back of the knee and ankle through its own tendons.

The plantaris muscle is basically a "pushing-off"

muscle—that is, it comes into use when you plant your foot and push off abruptly in a forward, or lateral, direction. Often, the long tendon connecting the lower end of the muscle to the heel will rupture during an excessive pushing-off maneuver or when you brace your leg to meet an oncoming force. This usually occurs at the point where the tendon and muscle blend together, just below the bulge of the calf, and when it does you will feel as though you have been whipped with a hot poker across the back of your calf.

Extreme pain follows. You will not be able to put your heel down and will be forced to limp around on the ball of your foot for sometime. As the rupture heals and the pain dissipates, your foot will remain in a heel-up position until you either have the taut tendon and muscle re-stretched manually or stretch it yourself through appropriate exercises.

Plantaris rupture is usually not a serious injury, but it can be quite disabling for several weeks if not attended to immediately. Early treatment should consist of the application of ice packs to the affected area, compression with an elastic bandage, and a heel lift on the shoe for two or three weeks. Later on, exercise will be necessary to rebuild the weakened muscle.

SHIN SPLINTS

This is an ailment common to all people who involve themselves in running sports, but is most frequently seen among joggers. It is an affliction whose nature is yet another source of confusion to many of its victims who believe it originates in the bones of their lower legs. It doesn't. Rather, it is an ailment of the anterior tibial muscles of the lower leg—three long, thin muscles that travel along the front of the leg, from below the knee to the foot, and function to lift the foot and, through their tendons, the toes.

Shin splints are basically a form of cramps in that they develop in a similar manner. When we run, especially on hard surfaces and after we have not done so for some time, the stresses on our unconditioned shin muscles are great. As they fatigue, they build up an oxygen debt and accumulate large amounts of lactic acid. When the debt becomes too much they go into spasm. The only difference between shin splints and ordinary cramps is that instead of going into acute spasms, the shin muscles develop milder but recurrent spasms. They become very hard, and when you touch the area it is difficult to tell the difference between the muscles and the lower-leg bone. As they become hard they act to squeeze off the veins, causing further engorgement and distention of the muscles.

The best way to deal with shin splints is to rest your legs until the pain and muscle hardness have disappeared. This generally takes one-to-two weeks. You can then resume running, but should do so gradually so that the shin muscles become properly conditioned over a period of time. It is not a bad idea, in addition, to wear knee-high socks to provide your shins with extra warmth. This stimulates blood supply to the areas and is one of the reasons so many professional basketball and football players wear them.

HAMSTRING PULLS

Your hamstring muscles are the long, thick muscles along the rear of your thigh that are the primary knee flexors. They too are highly prone to running injuries.

These injuries occur in the form of a tearing apart of muscle fibers, usually when sprinting, and can incapacitate the weekend athlete for weeks on end.

When we run at full speed, we exert tremendous pressures on our hamstring muscles as our knees travel rapidly through the flexion-extension process. When these muscles are weak or unconditioned, they often cannot stretch as far as our legs do. Like all muscles, when the stresses are repeated—as in a thirty- or forty-yard sprint in pursuit of a pop fly or long pass—the hamstrings can snap.

The sensation of a hamstring pull is similar to that of a plantaris rupture—it feels as though you have been thwacked across the back of your thigh with a hot poker. The fibers in the muscle will tear apart suddenly and you will pull up lame with an intensely searing pain. You will find further running impossible, and even walking will be difficult.

Again, this is not a serious ailment, but it can be discomforting for the eight-to-ten weeks it takes for a major tear to heal. The best way to deal with it is to allow it to heal through rest, and then proceed to recondition your hamstring muscles with stretching and strengthening exercises. Any exercise that puts a gradual stretching load on the backs of your thighs— even a simple toe-touch—is effective in making your hamstrings more supple. A good strengthening exercise is this:

Hold on to a doorknob, facing it, with your upper body bent slightly forward. Stand on one leg and let your other leg hang free. Swing your free leg forward, extending your knee; then slowly swing it backward and upward as far as you can. At the top of the arc, suddenly flex your knee so that the heel of your foot comes close to touching your buttocks. Repeat ten times, then switch to your other leg. When you have worked up to thirty easy repetitions for each leg, add ankle weights in two-pound increments.

GROIN PULLS

I have had more than a few patients ask me, "Doctor, what is this thing they call a 'groin' when they announce on television that such-and-such a player has a groin injury?" Others limp into my office certain they are the victims of hernias, only to discover they are merely suffering from a pulled groin muscle. We have here, then, another area of confusion.

The word "groin" describes nothing more than that area of the midline of the body where the thighs are joined to the torso. It might also be called the pubic region since the principal bones in the site are the pubic bones of the pelvis. Many people tend to think that only men have groins because "groin injury" is often used as a euphemism for an injury to the testicles. Not so—women possess groins too.

By a "groin pull" we mean a tear in one of the *hip adductor muscles*—those muscles that flow down along the interior of the hips and attach to the inner aspects of the thigh bone. Tears in these muscles usually come about because of sudden, intolerable adduction stresses, such as when one tries to close his or her thighs against a stronger opposite force, or when the legs are forced suddenly apart and the muscles are over-stretched.

Groin pulls are deep tears in the fibers of one of the

hip adductor muscles, either at the top of the inner thigh or on the lower pelvis itself. They can be worrisome and annoying, but are hardly ever serious. They can be prevented in all but the most stressful circumstances by conditioning and strengthening the groin muscles. Here are two good exercises to employ after a groin pull has healed:

1. Sit upright on the edge of a chair with a pillow clasped between your knees. Squeeze your knees together slowly against the pressure of the pillow, hold for a slow count of five, then relax. Repeat thirty times.

2. Stand with your legs widely separated. First bend one knee slowly to the floor, stretching the opposite adductor muscles. "Bounce" five times on your bent leg, and repeat on the other side.

SORE ARM

Probably the most common of all general muscle ailments is sore arm. Sore arm is simply a tear in the fibers of one of the muscles of the upper arm—usually the *biceps brachii,* which forms the principal muscle-mass along the forward aspect of the biceps, or the *brachialis,* which lies beneath the biceps, or the attachment of the deltoid. The cause is usually due to throwing, coupled with inherent weaknesses in the muscles themselves.

Once a sore arm develops, there is little that can be done for it except to allow the muscle to heal spontaneously, and then strengthen it through exercise.

This ailment tends to recur when throwing is resumed. Since it most probably came about as a result of throwing too hard without proper warm-up, it will recur under the same conditions. So the key to preventing its recurrence is to warm up your arm faithfully before ever trying to throw whatever it is you are throwing with any force. Of all muscle ailments, this is the one that is most frequently caused by an absence of common sense on the part of the sufferer. Thus, it will only be avoided in future by a plentiful infusion of common sense.

The range of general muscle ailments is far wider than space permits us to cover, but this brief discussion of the most frequent ones should give you a clear idea of their nature and mechanics. Muscle miseries—no matter where there site may be—develop out of a combination of direct and indirect causes. Direct causes are blows, strains, and stresses from without. Indirect causes are inherent weaknesses in unconditioned tissues and joints, and an inadequate oxygen supply within.

Many sports-related muscle ailments can be avoided with the exercise of a little knowledge and common sense. This is an entirely different form of exercising than physical exercises. Yet to achieve pain-free Mondays, it is an exercise you must pursue as diligently as you do your bodily pursuits.

13

A FINAL WORD

Your musculo-skeletal system is the foundation of all your activities—sports and otherwise. If it is not both strong and resilient, your ease and freedom of movement will be severely restricted, and your recreational athletic enthusiasms will be hindered.

Some injuries in sports are a natural hazard, we know. So are some ailments. But many could be avoided if their victims possessed flexible bodies. The key to a flexible body lies in the state of its connective tissues. Strengthening and enlarging the muscles is not all there is to physical fitness. Endurance and flexibility are equally important.

We've seen what can happen in our bodies when our muscles fatigue easily or fail to stretch properly to meet the needs of our athletic maneuvers. But muscles are just one kind of connective tissue. Ligaments, ten-

276

dons, cartilage, and other tissues also play an important role in holding your frame together. And we've seen what happens when these fatigue or fail to stretch.

Connective tissue, which is so liberally distributed throughout your body, has two major characteristics. First, it is *extensible*—that is, capable of being stretched. Second it is *compressible*—that is, it shortens when it is not in use.

The mobility of any of your joints is sustained by the fact that you use them all the time. If for some reason you don't use them (if your knee or shoulder is in a cast, for instance), the connective tissue around them compresses and movement becomes limited, stiff, and painful.

The standard treatment for a postoperative stiff joint is physical therapy—that is, gradual stretching. The connective tissue, which has shortened, must be elongated so that normal motion is once again possible. It only follows, then, that abnormal motion—such as occurs in many sports—requires *extra* extensibility. It is when that extensibility is not there at the time you need it that most miseries develop for the weekend athlete.

I said at the beginning of this book that I didn't put much stock in setting-up or calisthenic-type exercises as a way of maintaining physical fitness and endurance. Of course, any exercise is better than none. But if you are a weekend or part-time athlete, you would be much better advised to spend your time doing specific stretching and strengthening exercises than general calisthenics. Get your exercise from your sports activities, and use the time you usually devote to calisthenics to making your body more flexible so that you can get peak enjoyment and benefit from these activities.

Specific muscle-building exercises, such as those

I've outlined throughout this book, should be undertaken to strengthen and stretch specific muscles, but overall muscle development should not be your goal. Your objective should rather be to increase your body's overall resilience and flexibility. In addition, you should always warm up sufficiently before embarking on any athletic activity so that the flexibility of the joints and muscles that come under excessive strain in that activity will be enhanced and preserved.

With these prescriptions firmly rooted in your mind, you will find your weekend or recreational athletic endeavors producing fewer and fewer chronic miseries.

INDEX

INDEX

Abductor and abductor muscles,
   40–41
Aches:
   normal, 22
   reasons for, 15, 18
Achilles heel, 205
Achilles tendinitis, 208
Achilles tendon, 205–209
   exercises for, 209–210
   rupture of, 208
   surgery for, 208
Action-reaction, 49–50, 52–53
Aging, bone injuries and, 13
Ailments:
   ankle, 197–210
   athletics and, 23
   back, 155–196
   of ball-and-socket joint, 37
   body structure and, 24

diagnosis of, 4–5
foot, 251–260
hand and wrist, 238–250
hip, 227–237
knowledge of, 2
muscle, 261–275
prevention of, 1
psychology of, 2–3, 5
shoulder, 211–226
structural, 22
Ankle joint, 37, 41
Ankles, 251
   ailments of, 197–210
   braces for, 203
   exercises for, 203–204
   ligaments of, 197–201, 204
   muscles of, 203, 205
   sprained, 201–202
   weak, 201–205

281

Arm, 64, 75
    bones of, 212–213, 239
    sore, 274–275
    See also Forearm
Arm-and-shoulder pendulum
    exercise, 223
Arteries, 42–43
Arteriosclerosis, 43
Arthritis, 99
Arthrogram, 133
Aspirin, 86–87
Athletics, reasons for engaging
    in, 9–12

Back:
    ailments of, 155–156, 167–
        183
    bones of, 157–160
    chronic muscle strains in,
        187
    exercises for, 186–196
    knowledge of, 157–167
    ligaments of, 160–163
    muscles of, 31, 157, 163–
        167
    weak, 185–186
Back braces, 180, 182
Back injuries, 8
Back spasms, 176, 180–182
Backhand tennis stroke, 80,
        243–244
    ideal, 81
Baseball, 96–97
Baseball finger, 244–246
    treatment for, 245
Basketball, 144–146
Biceps, 64, 216–219
Biceps tendinitis, 219
Blood, 42
    insufficient supply of, 44,
        46–47
Blood clots, 43

Body:
    athletics and, 24
    complexity of, 23
    conditioning of, 15–16
    defense mechanisms of,
        12–13
    differences and sameness,
        23–24
    musculo-skeletal system of,
        26, 276
    personal knowledge of,
        25–55
Body line, 11
Bones, 26–28
    aging and, 13
    arm, 59–63, 65, 98, 212–
        213, 239
    back, 157–160
    characteristics of, 27–28
    of elbow, 59–61
    hand, 239
    hip, 228
    of knee, 106–108
    two components of, 26
    wrist, 249–250
Bowler's hip, 233
Bowler's thumb, 247–249
    treatment for, 249
Bowling, 248
Braces:
    ankle, 203
    back, 180, 182
    elbow, 91–92
Brain:
    action center of, 51
    nervous system and, 47, 49
Brain cells, 42
    muscle action and, 30
Bunions, 256–257
Bursae:
    hip, 231, 234–235
    inflammation of, 37, 231,
        235–236
    knee, 148–151

Bursitis, 37
    chronic, 220
    hip, 234–235
    patellar, 105
    shoulder, 219–223
Butazolidin treatment, 88–89

Calisthenics, 10–11, 277
Capillaries, 42
Capitulum, 59
Cartilages, 35–36
    articular, 108
    knee, 108–109, 116, 118–119, 125–126
    surgery for repair of, 132, 135
    torn, 104, 121, 132
Cells:
    brain, 30, 42
    nerve, 50–51
Cervical discs, 184–186
Charley horse, 262
Children:
    and little-league shoulder, 224–226
    and swimming, 265–266
Circulatory system, 42–47
Claw toes, 254–256
Coccyx region, 159
Conditioning, 79
    muscle, 17
Condyles, 106, 109
Connective tissue, 277
Corns, 257–258
Cortisone treatment, 87–89, 151, 219, 223, 232, 244
Cramps, 262–263
    heat, 265
    runner's, 264–265
    swimmer's, 265–268
Curveballs, 96

Dancer's knee, 105, 153–154
Dehydration, 12, 265
Doctors, 2–6
Doorway isometric exercise, 224
Dumbbells, 82, 100

Elbow braces, 91–92
Elbow joint, 37–40, 59, 101
    bony construction of, 59–61
    muscles and, 62–69
    tendons and, 65–66, 69
Embolus, 43
Epicondyles, 61, 78, 107
    lateral, 62–63, 66–70, 72–73, 75
    medial, 62–63, 94–95, 98, 101
    tissue damage and, 76
Exercise:
    benefits of, 11
    regular, 14
    sporadic, 11–12
    sports and, 9–11, 277
Exercises:
    ankle, 203–204
    back, 186–196
    elbow, 39
    and full-flexion joints, 39
    for groin pulls, 274
    for hamstring pulls, 272–273
    hip, 236–237
    for jumper's knee, 147
    knee, 38–39, 134–144, 147
    leg, 141–144
    muscle-building, 277–278
    shoulder, 223–224
    for slipped disc, 179, 181
    for sore arm, 275
    specific, 19, 21
    for tennis elbow, 81–84

for thrower's elbow, 99–101
for trick knee, 147
Exhaustion, 12
Extension motion, 39
Extensor muscles, 39, 64–70, 72,
  74–78, 81–82, 94, 96, 135,
  138, 164–166, 242

Fallen arches, 253–255
Fatigue fracture of foot bones,
  13
Feet:
  ailment of, 251–260
  arches of, 252–254
  bones of, 13, 251–253
  exercises for, 203–204
  flat, 253–254
Femur, 106, 108
Fibula, 106, 108, 110–111
Fingers, 239–240, 244–247
Flat feet, 253–254
Flexion motion, 39
Flexor muscles, 39, 74, 95–96,
  135, 140, 166, 242
Foot eversion exercise, 203–
  204
Foot inversion exercise, 204
Football, 8–9
Forearm, 64–65, 67–70
  development of, 74
  exercises for, 82–83
  muscles of, 73–75, 78, 101
Forearm extensor curl exercise,
  82–83
Forearm flexor curl exercise,
  100–101
Funny bone, 98

Gastrocnemii muscles, 136, 140,
  205, 269
Gibbs, Richard, 258
Golf, 234–235

Golfer's hip, 234–236
Gracilis muscle, 41
Groin pulls, 273–274
  exercises for, 274

Half sit-up exercise, 193, 195
Hammer toes, 254–255
Hamstring muscles, 136
Hamstring pulls, 271–273
  exercise for, 272–273
Hands, 68
  bones of, 239–240
  importance of, 238
  ligaments of, 240, 245
  muscles of, 242
  tendons of, 242
  wrists, and, ailments of,
    238–250
Heart, 42–43
Heat exhaustion, 12
Heat treatment, 223
Heel dip-and-raise exercise, 209
Hip abductor side-raise exercise, 236
Hip hyperextension exercise,
  195
Hip joint, 37, 40–41, 227
  bones of, 228
  ligaments of, 229
  muscles of, 229–233
Hip pointer, 231–232
  treatment of, 232
Hips:
  ailments of, 227–237
  exercises for, 236–237
  four basic motions of, 229
  muscles of, 165–167, 273–
    274
  pain and inflammation of,
    231–232, 235–236
Hospitalization for slipped disc,
  178, 180–181
Humerus, 59, 62–63, 212–213

Ice applications:
for baseball finger, 245
for hip pointer, 232
for tennis elbow, 86–87
Iliotibial band, 120, 131
Illness, prevention of, 7
Inflammation:
in bowler's thumb, 248
of bursae, 37, 231, 235–236
in hips, 231–233, 235–236
in jumper's knee, 144
of muscles, 261, 269
in swinger's wrist, 244
in tennis elbow, 67–68
in thrower's elbow, 101
in thrower's shoulder, 217
Injuries:
ankle, 201
back, 8
fatigue, 13
knee, 9, 19–22, 120–121
serious, 22–23
sports, 2, 78
Intervertebral disc, 169–171
Isometric forearm extension exercises, 83

Joints, 36–41, 62
ankle, 37, 41
ball-and-socket, 37, 40
cartilages and, 36
elbow, 37–40, 59, 62–69, 101
hinge, 37–41, 59, 66, 104, 109
knee, 36–39, 104–105, 148
ligaments and, 35
mobility of, 277
modified-hinge, 37, 41
muscles and, 39–41, 62–69, 261
stiff, treatment of, 277
wrist, 239

Jumper's knee, 105, 144–146
treatment, cure, and prevention of, 146–148

Knee-to-chest raise exercise, 189–190
Knee injuries, 9, 19–22, 121
Knee joint, 36–39, 102, 105
function of, 104
lubrication of, 148
Knee rotation exercise, 143–144
Kneecap, 138–139, 145, 148–149, 154
Kneeling, 149–150
Knees:
ailments of, 105–154
bones of, 106–108
cartilages of, 108–109, 116, 118–119, 125–126
dancer's, 153–154
dislocation of, 127 n.
displacement of, 127
injuries to, 9, 19–22, 120–121
jumper's, 105, 144–148
ligaments of, 33, 35, 104, 109–113, 116–125, 137–141
locked, 121–128
muscles of, 115, 135–143
painful, 102–103, 121
stresses on, 111, 116, 119–121, 124, 149
surfer's, 148–151
swollen, 19, 121
trick, *see* Trick knee
water on, 151–153

Lateral trunk stretch exercise, 191–192
Laver, Rod, 73
Leg swing exercise, 237

Legs:
    bones of, 13, 106–108, 112
    crossing of, 124–125
    exercises for, 134, 141–144
    muscles of, 261–274
Ligaments, 33–35
    of ankle, 197–202
    of back, 160–163
    function of, 35, 109
    of hand, 239, 245
    of knee, 33, 35, 104, 109–
       113, 116–125, 137–141
    ruptured, 129–131, 202
    shoulder, 214–216
    of spine, 35
    surgical repair of, 131, 135
    torn, 33, 104, 119, 121, 129–
       131, 202, 245
Little-league shoulder, 224–226
Locked knee, 121–126
    forward, 127
    rear, 127–128
    relaxation and, 128
    unlocking of, 126–128
Lower leg bones, 106–108, 112
Lumbago, 167, 174
Lumbar lordosis, 166, 171
Lungs, 42
    smoking and, 46

Mallet finger, 246–247
Medical terms, use of, 58
Muscle tone, 11
Muscles, 28–31
    abdominal, 164–165
    aching, 15
    ailments of, 261–275
    back, 31, 157, 163–167
    bruised, 269
    conditioning of, 17
    contraction of, 30, 40
    cramped, 262–268
    exercise and, 277–278

    fatigued, 276
    hip, 165–166, 273–274
    inflammation of, 261, 269
    interaction of, 64
    of joints, 39–41, 62–69, 261
    of knees, 115, 135–143
    nerves and, 28, 30
    shoulder, 214–217, 221–222
    skeletal, 28
    strained or pulled, 261,
       268–269, 271–274
    strengthening of, 79
    wrist and hand, 242
Musculo-skeletal system, 26, 276
Myelogram, 180, 182

Navicular fractures, 249–250
Neck, 158, 162
Nerve impingement, 97–99
Nerves, 47–48, 52–53
    damaged, 51
    median, 97–98
    motor, 49, 51–52
    radial, 97
    receptor, 51
    sensory, 49, 52–53
    ulnar, 94, 98–99
Nervous system, 47–51
    autonomic, 48
    somatic, 48–49
Neurological reflexes, 53–54
Newcombe, John, 71–72
Nose-to-knee touch exercise,
    193–194

Olecranon notch, 59, 61
Olecranon process, 61
Overactivity, 12
Oxygen:
    circulatory system and, 46
    muscles and, 30

Pain, 51–55, 168
   back, 163, 174–175, 178–182
   brain and, 53
   cortisone treatment for, 87–89, 151, 219, 223, 232, 244
   hip, 231–232, 235–236
   in knees, 102–105, 121
   nervous system and, 51–52
   normal, 22
   precipitating cause of, 53–54
   reasons for, 15, 18
   relief of, 85
   underlying cause of, 54
   variety of, 52
Patellar bursitis, 105
Patellar chondromalacia, 105
Patellar tendinitis, 105, 144–145
Pelvic tilt exercise, 190
Physical examinations, 12–13, 133
Pitchers, 96–97
Plantaris rupture, 269–270
Poor posture, 166
Professional athletes, 79, 97
Pronator muscle, 67–68, 70, 74, 94

Quadriceps extensor raise exercise, 141–142
Quadriceps muscles, 20–21, 136–138, 140–142

Radius, 59–60, 62, 65
Reed, Willis, 144
Rest treatment, 77, 86–87, 147, 151, 177–179, 181, 209, 219, 223, 232, 244, 270, 272

Rotator cuff muscles, 216, 220–222
Runner's cramps, 264–265

Sacrum, 159
Saddle joint, 37, 41
Scapula, 212–213
Sciatica, 167, 174
Scissors exercise, 194–195
Screwballs, 96
Setting-up exercises, 17–18
Shin splints, 270–271
Shoes, 257, 259
   tennis, 258–259
Short-windedness, smoking and, 46
Shoulder, 75
   ailments of, 211–216
   basic anatomy of, 212–216
   dislocated, 215
   exercises for, 223–224
   separated, 215
Shoulder bursitis, 219–223
   treatment of, 223
Shoulder joint, 37, 40–41, 65, 211, 213
   ligaments of, 214–216
   muscles of, 214–216, 221–222
   tendons of, 215
Side-and-front arm raise exercise, 224
Single straight-leg raise exercise, 192–193
Skater's ankles, 201–205
Skier's heel, 205–209
Skiing, 205–207, 219, 222
Slipped disc, 167–175
   surgery for, 183–184
   treatment of, 175–183
Smoking, 46–47
Softball, 96
Sore arm, 274–275

Spinal column, 172
Spinal cord, 161
Spinal discs:
    cervical, 184–186
    protruded, 173, 177–178
    ruptured, 173
    slipped, *see* Slipped disc
    stretched or pulled, 176
Spine, 157–165, 167–168
    four curves of, 171
    four regions of, 158–159
    ligaments of, 35
Sports:
    competitive, 10
    participation in, 1–3, 10–11,
        13
    and specific ailments, 22
    strenuous, caution about,
        12–14
    weekend, 14–22
    See also names of sports
Sports-medicine, 3–4
Sprinter's stretch exercise, 236–
    237
Stiffness, reasons for, 15, 18
Straight-leg abductor exercise,
    143
Straight-leg raise exercise, 143
Sunstroke, 12
Supinator muscle, 67–68, 70, 74,
    94
Surfer's knee, 105, 148–151
    causes of, 150
    treatment of, 151
Surfer's knobs, 151
Surgery:
    for Achilles tendon, 208
    for bunions, 257
    for jumper's knee, 147
    to repair torn cartilages,
        132, 135
    for slipped disc, 183–184
    for tennis elbow, 90–91
    for trick knee, 147
Swayback, 166

Swimmer's cramps, 265–268
Swimming, 219, 265–268
Swinger's wrist, 243–244
Symptoms, treatment of, 5
Synovium, 152

Tendinitis, 224
    Achilles, 208
    biceps, 219
    patellar, 105, 144–145
Tendons, 31–33, 65–66, 69, 76
    Achilles, 205–210
    patellar, 145–147
    quadriceps, 137, 149
    shoulder, 215
    wrist and hand, 241–242,
        247
Tennis, 12, 15, 218, 243
    body power used in, 75
    hitting backhand in, 80
Tennis ball, constant hitting of,
    70
Tennis ball squeeze exercise,
    83
Tennis elbow, 18, 56, 95, 244
    effects of, 75–77
    exercises for, 82–84
    inflammation and, 67–68,
        75–77, 85
    medical term for, 58, 67
    precipitating causes of, 57,
        69–73
    prevention of, 78
    among recreational players,
        71
    sources of, 57–58
    spontaneous remission of,
        92–93
    surgery for, 90–91
    treatment of, 77–79, 82–89
    underlying causes of, 73–
        75
Tennis rackets, 87
Tennis shoes, 258–259

Tennis shoulder, 215–219
Tennis stroke:
    body position in, 80–81
    ideal, 71
    improper, 72, 75–76
    proper, 71–72, 75, 79
Tennis toe, 258–259
Thigh bone, 106, 112
Thrombophlebitis, 45
Throwers, 96–97
Thrower's elbow, 93–97
    causes of, 94
    medical term for, 94
    nerve impingement and, 97–99
    treatment of, 99–101
Thrower's shoulder, 215–219
    treatment for, 219
Thumb, 247–249
Thumb joint, 37
Tibia, 106–108, 110, 148
Tissues, 97
    conditioning of, 17
Toes, 254–260
Touch football, 19–21
Traction for slipped disc, 179
Treatment:
    of bowler's thumb, 249
    butazolidin, 88–89
    cortisone, *see* Cortisone treatment
    heat, 223
    of hip pointer, 232
    by ice application, 86–87, 232, 245
    of jumper's knee, 146–148
    objectives of, 86–87
    rest, *see* Rest treatment
    of shoulder bursitis, 223
    for slipped disc, 175–183
    of surfer's knee, 151
    of symptoms, 5
    of tennis elbow, 77–79, 82–89
    of thrower's elbow, 99–101

of thrower's shoulder, 219
of trick knee, 133–144
Triceps, 64
Trick knee, 19–21, 30, 33, 103–104
    causes of, 114–115
    collapsing, 122
    exercises for, 134–144
    ligaments and, 116–125
    management of, 133–144
    mechanics of, 116–126
    surgery for, 131–135
    X ray of, 133
Trochlea, 59, 61

Ulna, 59, 61–63, 65, 98
Upper arm, 64, 75

Veins, 42–43
    breakdown of, 45
    varicose, 45
Vertebrae, 157–159
Volleyball, 144–146

Wall bounce exercise, 209–210
Warm-up, 97, 101
Water on the knee, 151–153
Weekend athletes, 14, 97
    abnormal miseries of, 18–22
    hazards of, 78
    normal miseries of, 14–18
Whiplash, 162
Wrist, 65, 67–68, 70, 75, 94–95
    bones of, 249–250
    and hands, ailments of, 238–250
    joints of, 239
    tendons of, 241–242, 247

X rays, 133, 180, 181, 226, 245